Jeffrey S. Hakes

Holy. War.

How I Ended My Affair With Porn

and fell in love with Jesus

Holy. War. How I Ended My Affair with Porn and Fell in Love with Jesus.

ISBN 978-0-578-80005-9

Introduction

Don't get me wrong: I'm not a crier, by any means. But I must confess, I've been known to wipe tears from my eyes during the showing of movie trailers. No, not the chick-flick romantic ones. Nor those intense dramas where someone is struggling with cancer or divorce or whatever. No—tears come to me from scenes of battle-field conflict between good and evil.

Writing in early 2019, I teared up during a Mulan trailer (!), and the trailer for the upcoming, Midway. Years earlier, tears found my cheeks during the showing of the film, the Matrix, during the Bourne Identity series, and while watching The Edge Of Tomorrow. I suddenly broke into tears when King Peter raised his sword and his voice and led the charge against the White Witch's forces in the battle for Narnia's liberation in the Lion, the Witch, and the Wardrobe.

The tears I experience in theaters are always unexpected, and almost always, if they come, they threaten to undo me. You see, I have within me both a profound longing for battle, and a solid memory of the nightmare of former enslavement. In trying to understand this peculiarity of mine, I have come to see that I cry at such scenes in movies because I know what it is like to have been a tormented prisoner, to have lived under a cruel, lying tyrant, to have been betrayed, and deceived, dominated, and to have longed and prayed for a deliverer. I cry now because, having been rescued, I know I am called to help rescue others, to see oppression and the dominion of darkness ended, to see trafficked human souls set free. As long as there remain those who are searching for the freedom like I drink deeply from daily, I am surrendered passionately to handing out road maps to true liberation.

You see, I can't wait to see the devil go to Hell. And until he does, crushed under my feet by the God of Peace, I want to lend a strong hand and my sword to those who want to escape the effects of darkness.

This book is my earnest effort to create just that, and place the truth-empowered keys of supernatural deliverance within reach of someone who—despite their best, valiant efforts and intentions for change— is finding that their *will* is somehow still enslaved, as mine was, through entanglement with pornography.

Porn stole well over 15 years from me and my family. Although they have healed well, the mistakes I made have left scars that will walk with me through the rest of my life. Before that healing came, for years I searched for help. I fasted and prayed for help. And I even asked several christian professionals for the help I needed. But those I asked were unaware of the mechanics of what I was dealing with, particularly ignorant of the supernatural dimension fueling the battle for my heart. So their answers were ineffective in producing lasting transformation. Some of those I went to for help even outright condemned me; but someone else pointed me toward a very down-to-earth social worker that was unafraid to take my case; His name was Jesus. He told me He had been already searching for me, and that His purpose was to destroy the work of the devil in my life. Once I started to listen to the voice of this Wonderful Counselor, my eyes were opened to the supernatural dimension of my struggle, and the decisive way out of the forest I was so lost in was no longer hard to find.

By the scandalous grace of God and the choice of my own free will, I have walked in freedom from my addiction to pornographic deception for 20 years now. Ever since my deliverance, I have felt this haunting sense that there must be others like I was, people searching desperately for someone who knows a way out of the labyrinth, someone who can unplug the powers of darkness that masquerade behind the airbrushed pawns of pornography. I am sure there are millions who have been so liberated; I certainly do not have the corner on this insight, and so have put off writing this book for two decades. But I now feel compelled by the passionate Holy Spirit to share my story.

If you are among those hunting for effective, supernatural answers to the question of how to stop your engagement with porn, then take hope: I truly believe that what brought lasting salvation to me is transferable to you. Alarmed by the increase of pornography in the church, and challenged by the passionate Holy Spirit to personally play a larger role in turning those tables, I felt I must do what I can to make my story available to you, in case what I have learned is exactly the combination of things you need to know in order to pick the lock on your chains and step out into the fullness of life beyond pornographic intimacy.

We overcome by the blood of the Lamb and the word of our testimony. I have written here 15 testimonial chapters, each of which contain a step God invited me to take as He walked me out of my deception and into the Truth that set me free. They are all full of scripture and record words the Spirit of God spoke to me to lead me into freedom. You might want to read one chapter a day for 15 days straight, slowly digesting what I am proposing. What you will find is not academia, not psychology. These are not mental concepts, nor strictly intellectual information. Instead, what I have tried to do is re-present to you details from the encounters I had with the God who chased after me, found me, and instructed my change. They will challenge your mind; you will need to taste them with your spirit. Meditate on them. Ask the Holy Spirit to help you taste of the good things that He set on the table for me, in the very presence of my enemies. In so doing, I am sure you will see as well that the Lord is good.

Understand that I am in not only interested in seeing you walk in the fullest possible freedom from a repetitive sin cycle. I am as well interested in seeing you go beyond such deliverance, to see you step into the effervescent offer of actually participating in life the life of Christ, walking out your remaining days in the wonderful, exuberant embrace of holiness. It is for such FREEDOM that you have been set free! That is the truth. Beyond the choking effects of addiction to porn, there is a life of transcendent purpose, and a fountain of creativity, as you enter into the poetry of things already prepared and waiting for you and God to do together.

This book will offer you a new day and a new opportunity. It will place before you the truth of life or death and require you to make an informed choice. I pray especially that you will take up its invitation to the liberation of your own will and to the surrender of it to the only intimacy that truly satisfies.

Chapter Index

Dedication:

With endless gratitude to my priceless, undaunted, heaven-focused Caryn Beth, whose transfusions of courageous, sacrificial love revived my heart

For our truly luminous son and daughter, Austin Jacob and Rachel Anne, and their stellar spouses, Amanda Caitlin and Brian Keith, so you all could know the storm and the calm that followed

Acknowledgements:

The insight, honesty, and artistry of the Foreman brothers and their amazing band, Switchfoot, have deeply impacted my life and cheered on my faith for twenty years of international ministry. Love *IS* a movement.

I am forever grateful for Dr. Neil Anderson, whose books skillfully pointed me to Jesus, who pointed me to freedom.

Chapter 1 The Naked Truth

November, 1997

As was often the case in Nairobi, perched just south of the equator, the day was dressed in steam and pungent, unexplainable odor. Even with the morning still young, under the untamed African sun, sweat surfed down my spine, soaking my cotton shirt and jeans as I reigned the Toyota Hiace van through the fish-school of heavy traffic already overwhelming the streets of this sprawling city of five and a half million. Two cups of bitter Kenyan coffee down, my hands vice-gripped the wheel, sun-glassed eyes ever darting: whenever I was in the capital city, I determined to remain hyper-focused, on my guard against being swept away in its churning volatility.

At the time, I was the purchasing agent for a large mission school and outpost infirmary located an hour away in the mountains that overlook the Great Rift Valley. This particular Thursday morning, I was heading into the bowels of the city, where I would invest hours in negotiating for office supplies, bulk food, medicines, tools, whatever was on the list given to me to secure for the continued operation of the mission station I represented.

My responsibilities also included currency exchange for the foreign staff; often my briefcase, and the pockets of my cargo pants—sometimes even my socks— were stuffed full of several currencies—US and Canadian dollars, British Pounds, South African Rand, and Kenyan Shillings— as I navigated the disarray of Nairobi's tangled streets, where violent crime was increasingly a part of the makeup of the city. On the job, I was appropriately nervous, wide awake, and all eyes.

Among the labyrinthine backstreets of the bustling industrial zone, I had made several stops already that morning and loaded cases of supplies into the cargo bay of the van. After checking my "to-do" list again, I pulled into the parking lot in front of what was a new stop for me, in order to pick up some automotive parts the school's mechanic had ordered. Especially alert in this new environment, chin up to dismiss any outward sign of vulnerability, I strode purposefully into the large shop. Underneath the galvanized roofing that spread its sheltering wings perhaps 30 feet overhead, the service counter stretched 50 feet wide, inviting many customers to be attended to at the same time by the several Indian merchants who stood at attention between the counter and the rows of shelving, holding automotive parts from companies all over the world. All this my eyes took in in an instant before they were completely arrested by a towering naked female figure.

Sentry-like, a round marble pillar stood at each end of the room, rising all the way to carry the supporting rafters just under the steel roofing sheets above. The pillars themselves were impressive, both their oversized strength and lavish beauty out of place in the otherwise austere, strictly function-oriented, third world warehouse and sales depot. However, what caught my attention was not so much the marble pillars themselves, but what they were adorned with: each of them bore the full-color, 20 foot tall photographic display of an Indian woman of extraordinary beauty, "dressed" in an almost entirely see-through gauze. The roundness of each pillar the woman was displayed on only added an element of 3D, making her appear almost real. Her riveting, deep brown-eyed gaze was entrancing, her smirk enticing, and the transparent fabric that wrapped her upper torso left nothing to the imagination. The gauze then wafted strategically past the tender region below her waist, obscuring genitalia but displaying the perfect curve of her hips, the pillars of her legs, the graceful plant of her jeweled feet.

The display. was. stunning.

Do you really want to engage in idolatry?

Pornography is illegal in Kenya. In my then six years of work in East Africa, I had never seen any public display of pornography, nor even a commercial outlet where porn magazines were among the offerings. I'd have to say that beyond Kenya, in all my years in fact, I had never seen a naked woman who stood fully twenty feet tall! As I think back on the scene now, it was actually the immense height of the woman that broke through reality to stun my gray matter with a profound spiritual revelation: instead of seeing her as a naked *woman*, I saw her as she was, even as I heard myself unexpectedly mouth the words aloud:

"This is not a photo of a woman: this is an idol!"

Still hyper-alert to security concerns and the related danger of distraction, I processed that sentence at lightning speed. With certainty, although I had never before considered *pornography* in connection to *idolatry*, in my heart I was immediately aware that what I was seeing was not only a display of natural, God-designed, transcendent beauty; I was being informed that His excellent design had been hijacked, leaving before me a supernaturally empowered invitation to the capture of one's attention, the worship of something else, something dark, something powerful and larger than life.

Hmmmm . . .

I was not at all accustomed to "hearing the voice of God" at the time, but in my arrested reflection that morning I recall hearing instantly the inquiry, and knowing that it came from Heaven:

"Are you an idolater?"

There was no accusation in the gentle question, just an invitation to honest introspection and a search for the truth. I was silent, confused, so the Questioner took a new approach and whispered to my mind again:

"Do you want to engage in idolatry?"

When faced with *that* question, I found the answer quickly, and my heart readily confessed:

"NO— of course not!"

I was left then in silence, still standing between the two pillars. The absence of further communication from heaven seemed to confirm that there was nothing more to discuss: the brazen, towering nudity on either side of me had been clearly, divinely identified as idolatrous; having identified it as such, I had been wordlessly counseled to have nothing to do with it, regardless of its attractive powers. End of discussion.

So I moved confidently to the counter, ordered the parts on my list, waited with unswerving gaze for my items to be brought to me, paid the bill, turned and walked straight back to my waiting van, without the slightest second glance at the gods of that establishment.

Surprisingly, after years of my grappling alone with pornography and bearing its related shame and terror, and after my long, fruitless, frustrating search for help to make sense of my impotence on this battle ground, it was this unexpected, directly supernatural encounter one steamy Kenyan morning that was the beginning of my long-awaited deliverance from the power of porn.

Genesis of my obsession

Let's jump into this; my own struggle with sexual sin was in reference to its sense of dominion over my will. At the time, I found sexual sin—specifically exposure to nudity—absolutely fascinating, and at times found myself incapable of saying "no" to its invitation. Having been born spiritually when I was 16, as I began to grow in my personal, relationship-with-God based faith, I found this struggle of my will over the power of porn very disconcerting, at times horrifying, and I began to search for help with winning the battle for my will that I found myself too often engaged in.

Here's a brief history of the genesis of my struggle: as an eight-year-old, I began to be pursued by an age-mate I'll call Verona. She was a very attractive young girl, with a bubbling personality, an engaging smile, and glistening blond hair. Daughter of a large family in our community, she seemed in many ways to be a normal, healthy youngster, but Verona was profoundly troubled—someone had exposed her to adult sexual activity. And so Verona began to insist that we repeat this "grown up" behavior in our own friendship.

Almost from the first private conversation she had with me (at an organized church youth function at the local roller skating rink) as an eight year old, she expressed direct interest in having intimacy with me (not that those were her words). I had no concept at all of what she was talking about, but she kept asking me to "make out" with her. Again, we were eight-years-old. So I replied then as probably most any healthy eight-year-old boy would: I told her an emphatic and disgusted "no!"

It took years of her consistently pursuing me before I gave in to her pressure, and I began, on a dare, to interact with her physically, almost against my will at first and with a complete lack of interest on my part at the time. Entirely under her direction, almost instantly we went from holding hands to oral sexual contact, all of which was completely alien to me and brought absolutely no arousal to my young body. That did not seem to matter to her. She was determined to force me to experience what someone else had forced her to experience. Without anyone's knowledge but our own, years of intense physical intimacy followed, during which, in time, my own awakening to sexual interest eventually took place.

During this time, our interactions could best be described as having no personal relational base. Still children really, we were not interested in, or even yet very capable of a personal relationship. Sadly, like animals under the influence of seasonal scent on the wind, we were somehow captivated by the power of mindless sexuality. We remained interactive from the time I was eleven or twelve until late in my fifteenth year.

My mid-teenage years brought a change to me, as I slowly began to grow into and develop the natural capacity for personal interaction and relationships. On God's time clock, I had my first wet dream as a fourteen-year-old. On God's time clock, I slowly began to take a genuine interest in girls for the beauty of who they were —that part of His own image that He deliberately encased only in the female. The mystery and wonder of contemplating friendship over the cross-cultural dividing lines of boy/girl began to dawn on me in a holy fashion. At the same time, I had this awakening spiritual call, and with it a hunger for what was pure and right. As I matured, I began to see that what Verona offered was no longer tasteful to me. I suppose it was simply by God's grace, with no one else's guidance or assistance, that I was able to walk entirely away from interacting with Verona.

Although it would have been tremendous for me to have entered that sacred arena of my teenage years in a healthy state, in reality, by then I had a strongly developed double-mindedness—publicly, I was a good little boy who hardly ever got into any trouble, while privately I was engaged in a darkly empowered, riveting fascination with sex.

Let's skip the sad and sordid details and jump to later in the story. Although Verona became a thing of my past, even as I was born again at 16, during my mid-teens insatiable hunger for the tremendous pleasures she'd awakened of sexual stimulation opened doors to experimentation with pornography and eventually with masturbation.

New doors, new darkness

Let me introduce an invented term here: *Pornographic Intercourse*. Pornographic intercourse {a term I am creating here for the sake of our discussion} is the use of pornography (or other illicit visual sexual stimuli) coupled with masturbation for the purpose and end of achieving sexual climax. As I walked away from the sexual abuse

Verona had engaged me with, pornographic intercourse eventually became a cyclical part of my life.

I never discussed with anyone at the time the strange relationship I had had with Verona, nor any of the sexual volatility I was carrying in the wake of my relationship with her. Instead, as time went on, I dragged those dark, unprocessed secrets on into my life, through my late teen years, through my college years, and eventually into the otherwise happy marriage and young family I had started. I still cannot contemplate without terrible shame the depths I'd stoop to, during this particularly dark period, in order to find brief satisfaction for the crazed, cyclical sexual hunger that was launched like a virus in me as a child. But I will say that I began to realize that I needed help.

What I felt by the time that I was in my late twenties was that there was something dark in me that I could not control, a tremendous, ravenous hunger, unhealthy, unmanageable. I slowly came to the awareness that pretty much my every thought of every woman who crossed my path on any given day was to objectify them, to consider their value only in terms of them as sexual entities, to look them over lustfully in an effort to satisfy an internal hunger that I now know was a longing to know and to be known, a longing for union.

By now I was the husband of a deeply beautiful, godly woman, the father of a young son and a new baby girl; I was holding down two jobs, working seven days a week to provide us with a lower middle class income. We had a nice enough home and things looked okay from the outside. But inside I was a mess; sexual misconduct was a growing secret and private hell that began to break my mind. I was, as the Bible states, *". . . a double-minded man, unstable in all his ways"* (James 1:8). In desperation and rising concern, I can recall beginning to cry out to God for help. "Please take these desires away from me!" This became my almost constant prayer. Bound to His sacred commitment not to violate my own free will, God was not eager to give me what I was asking for.

In the mid-eighties, there was a sudden new buzzword in the evangelical conservative circles we were a part of at the time: *accountability groups*. Hopeful, I deliberately joined an "accountability" group in the mega-church we attended, hoping that it would be the silver-bullet answer to my private war. It was not. I went faithfully to all the meetings and interacted as openly and honestly as I could each week; the three other guys in our cell group were highly educated, very wealthy professionals; I was a truck driver and public school night shift custodian. Although it did not need to be an obstacle, the educational and career mismatch wasn't exactly grounds for deep, connective friendship. Still, I thought these other men might help me;

but before confessing anything deep, I kept waiting to be asked by the three others in the group the personal questions that would open the doors to help for me. None were ever asked. I'm not sure why, but there was never any real attempt at all by anyone in the group to *get to know me*, much less to become comrades in the fight for my much-needed deliverance from the power of sexual sin. The relationally shallow waters of the group, plus my own hesitation to engage in honest disclosure, ensured I'd have to look elsewhere for my silver bullet.

Searching for rescue

So I took it to the next level: I went to our church's pastoral counselor. This time I was more forward with my issues, knowing I needed and really wanted help. I confessed to the Pastor my struggle with pornography and my desire to see its' power broken. I remember that he was very compassionate and made quick work of making sure I did not feel so badly about myself. With great confidence and a fatherly, condescending smile, he gently redirected my attention: "What I think is your *real* struggle is that you need to be more self-actualized." He then recommended I see a professional Christian Psychologist, someone I'll call here Dr. Rolf, also a member of the church.

So I contacted this highly respected Christian counselor— a Doctor in Psychology this time— and made an appointment. Again I was very forward with my issues, eager for help. For the second time, teary-eyed, shame-wrapped, I confessed my struggle with pornography and my desire to see its power broken. This counselor was also very compassionate and again made quick work of making sure I did not feel so badly about myself. As if reading from the script of the previous Pastor's advice, this psychologist also responded with great confidence and a fatherly, condescending smile, and gently redirected my attention to what he believed was really my problem: "What I think is your *real* struggle is that you need to be more self-actualized."

While I remain grateful for the compassionate efforts of these gentlemen, I still shake my head at such a misguided response. Here's why: *natural remedies cannot ever hope to effectively treat a problem that has a supernatural foundation!* Let me explain . . .

When Jesus was first confronted with the case of the Maniac of Gadera, imagine that after His first initial inquiry of the naked demoniac, Jesus explained gently that what this guy *really* needed was to be more self-actualized. To have given him such an answer would have been to leave him bound to darkness, and only further, more deeply frustrated in his own best efforts to find freedom and health. Granted, I was not a host to a demonic legion. But I was far enough into this mess that even I could sense there was a supernatural strength to my problem. Hearing that what I needed was mere personal development made no sense to me: I cannot tell you how frustrated I was by this time. I knew I was carrying darkness around in me, battling addiction. I needed deliverance. But those to whom I turned only tried to help me feel better about myself.

Needless to say, after several sessions, none of which addressed sexuality (or sin) *at all*, and for which this time I had to pay good money, I stopped going to see Dr. Rolf.

In 1992, in spite of still-buried secret struggles, I was beginning a move into honest spiritual development and maturity, spurred on by my wife's tremendous walk of faith, and inspired by things like the trendy book, The Ragamuffin Gospel, author Brennan Manning's hopeful treatise on the overwhelming grace and love of God in the face of our marked propensity for stumbling faith. Maybe there was hope for me after all, I mused.

A year later, after selling our home and taking a great leap of faith by answering an invitation to direct involvement in world missions, we moved our young family to Kenya where, as mentioned, I became the purchasing agent (and dorm parent, high school shop teacher, and director of security) for a mission outpost in the mountains. I was really taking great strides toward spiritual growth and personal maturity, but I was still battling the ghosts of my past and was looking for the help I had not yet found. So again, this time as a missionary on the foreign field, I sought out a licensed christian psychologist there in Kenya. Again I confessed my sin and longing for help. This time the gravity of my error seemed to sink in with the counselor. He was honestly concerned. But I recall he offered no hope, no help, no counsel. He responded with an attitude of judgement and ambivalence, moving away from me instead of reaching out to help me. Further isolated and humiliated, I left his office after just one visit and soldiered on alone, continuing to cry out to God for help.

For the next several years on the mission field, although now very sincerely involved in both personal spiritual growth and fruitful ministry on many sides, I also continued to struggle in silence and isolation with secrets inside. The battle was tremendous: I really wanted to be a good husband, a good father, a good Christian and leader; alone, I fought with all the personal nobility I could round up. But occasionally—maybe only 3 or 4 times in 12 months—my resolve would break under the insanity that seemed to flow through my mind, and I would sneak money out of our personal budget, and while in Nairobi, purchase pornography at black market outlets, and engage in pornographic intercourse.

The ugly face behind the mask

It was in late 1997, after several unsuccessful attempts to get professional help in dealing with this struggle, that I had that encounter with the 20 foot tall "idols" at the automotive shop. Let me explain the impact of this event.

Behind the complexities of pornographic intercourse there are intricate mental gymnastics that must be dealt with very seriously— mind games, illusions, and lies that can only be properly dismantled with the help of the Holy Spirit. I believed and have experienced the intricacies of lie upon lie upon lie that weave a shield over the eyes of one's understanding, so that the participant in an addictive cycle of behavior is almost entirely ignorant of the compromise of character that addictive sin requires of its victim. The sudden, public exposure to me of a beautiful 20' tall nude woman that day at the parts shop in Nairobi brought such a shock to my spirit that for a moment, the mask of physical beauty that I was accustomed to gazing on and bowing to (and had been bowing to ever since I first said "yes" to Verona) slipped, and I saw behind it the ugly face of Darkness, directly orchestrating, redirecting, and demanding my fascination. For a fraction of a moment, I did not see a naked woman; I "saw" (or understood that what I was really seeing was) a naked demon, a fallen angel, the devil, *whatever*. I'm not going to get too hung up on exactly *what* I saw, but as it was standing there so starkly identified by God *as an Idol*, stripped of its makeup, I did not find the devil's mask so attractive; and so for the first time, I was able to turn away and say "no" to pornography. That was my first real step toward deliverance.

Chapter 2 The First and Greatest Wound

Idolatry. Webster's defines idolatry as: "the worship of a physical object as a god." I would venture to guess that in this strict sense, idolatry is probably not a topic you've given a lot of thought to in today's Western society. Perhaps if you really looked for them, you might find locations even in America where people go to formally worship idols, that is, to bow down to a physical object or statue as if it were a real god. In Wikipedia there is an article on idolatry that includes the following: "In many Indian religions, such as theistic and non-theistic forms of Hinduism, Buddhism, and Jainism, idols are considered as symbolism for the absolute . . . or icons of spiritual ideas, or the embodiment of the divine. (An idol) is a means to focus one's religious pursuits and worship. In the traditional religions of ancient Egypt, Greece, Rome, Africa, Asia, the Americas and elsewhere, the reverence of an image or statue has been a common practice, and cult images have carried different meanings and significance."

Having been raised in upstate New York in a strict conservative home, the only cult image-type of idolatry I had been exposed to was that which one encounters in the reading of the Bible. Idolatry gets a lot of press in the pages of scripture, from its stark prohibition in the Ten Commandments, to the major part it plays as an ongoing distraction for the children of Israel in their attempt to live their divine calling to be a Kingdom of priests, set apart from the practices of the world, devoted instead purely to the worship of God. Scripture is clear: idols are forbidden!

Surely I had not ever been involved in (or even considered the possibility of being attracted to) the worship of an image or statue. Yet standing at the auto parts counter in Nairobi, the Holy Spirit had clearly identified the towering nudity on display as *idolatry*, and asked me if I was an *idolater*.

A couple of valuable questions came to mind there: How could that pornographic display be an idol? And how could my gazing at it have been in any way connected to worship?

Pondering these questions on my own, I decided to head into scripture to find out.

DNA of Idolatry

Let's start with the original mention of what later is formally labeled as idolatry. In Exodus chapter 20, verses1-6, we find the following under the heading, The Ten Commandments:

"And God spoke all these words, saying: 'I am the Lord your God, who brought you out of the land of Egypt, out of the house of bondage.

'You shall have no other gods before Me.

'You shall not make for yourself a carved image—any likeness of anything that is in heaven above, or that is in the earth beneath, or that is in the water under the earth;

'You shall not bow down to them nor serve them. For I, the Lord your God, am a jealous God, visiting the iniquity of the fathers upon the children to the third and fourth generations of those who hate Me, but showing mercy to thousands, to those who love Me and keep My commandments.'"

Without taking too much time on this point, it is my opinion that what God is saying in the presentation of these first two commands is this:

"(Always remember:) I am the One who delivered you from abject slavery, thereby creating a special, transcendent people group out of a class of former slaves. You were drones; but now you are all royal children. You were purposeless; now you are highly purposed. On the basis of

that as your understanding of Me as Redeemer and you as Redeemed, I alone must be the primary object of the affections of your heart, of your adoration, your bowing down in worship and of your service. I really am the only safe direction for your capacity for fascination, the direction of your attention. Making an image of something else and bowing down to it as if It were your Redeemer is something that I explicitly prohibit; if you choose to do so, I will respond in passionate jealousy and I will interpret your actions as rejection—as actual hatred—of Me."

"Furthermore, your choosing to make an image to bow down and serve as a god instead of Me is so serious in My sight that it will result in a curse being released into your family lines, for three or four generations.

"On the other hand, your choice to obey this command translates into your loving Me; and I will respond to that choice by blessing a thousand generations of those who so obey and love Me."

At its core foundation, I suggest that worship of the God of Abraham, Isaac, and Jacob is choosing to appropriately contemplate and respond to the gift of liberation from slavery; *at its foundation, the appropriate response to the gift of Redemption is acknowledgement of the Redeemer as the One who alone is capable of truly satisfying one's every need.*

With this definition as a backdrop for further contemplation, I propose then that *idolatry is choosing instead to turn away from the offering of the Redeemer, and to return to a mindset and lifestyle of enslavement to a false offer of succor from any other venue.*

The Reality at Porn's Core

As I contemplated this, I sensed that the Spirit of God was saying that the pornographic display I'd encountered in Kenya was not so much about *sexuality* as it was about *idolatry;* this is a very important consideration. It's one thing to consider that in my casually engaging in pornographic intercourse, I might be doing something vaguely wrong; it's another thing entirely to have that vague wrongdoing suddenly defined by God as idolatry, and my involvement in it as the breaking of the first and greatest commandment, and the wounding of the very heart of God.

With God's Spirit coaching me, I began to contemplate idolatry—a sin I had previously relegated to *other* people in *other* countries where people bow down to statues— in an entirely different light, realizing for the first time that idolatry may be something that *I* might be guilty of having engaged in. I began to read scriptures about idolatry in a different manner, and in so doing, my own heart began to break as I thought, perhaps for the first time really, about the tender heart and feelings of God.

{This, in fact, is one of the chief aims of this manuscript: to invite you to contemplate with me the heart of God, no longer as One infinitely removed from our experience, no longer as stoic, unfeeling, invulnerable, unmoved, incapable of personal injury; God is inviting us—requiring us in fact— to contemplate His heart as the tender heart of a loving *Husband*. Please stop for a moment and ask the Holy Spirit to give you a revelation of God as Husband as you continue to read; of course, the echo to such contemplation is the consideration of yourself as the focus of His husbandly affection. This revelation too will be an important part of your deliverance from bondage to the false intimacy of pornographic intercourse.}

Heaven's Bride

Although the thought might be foreign to many western Christians, focused as they are on New Testament texts about the Bride of Christ, Israel is actually clearly referred to in many scriptures as the wife of God. Examples abound:

". . .Return to me . . . for I (God) am married to you (Israel)." (Jer. 3:14)

" . . . For your maker is your (Israel's) husband."
(Isaiah 54:5a)

Perhaps the most touching of these obviously allegorical husband/bride references (and there are *many*) is found in Ezekiel 16. The whole of this long, must-read chapter unfolds like the script of a tragic romance drama. It starts out with God out for a walk and encountering an infant, tossed into a field to die on its own: *" . . . when I passed by you and saw you struggling in your own blood, I said to you . . . 'Live!' Yes, I said to you in your blood, 'Live!' I made you thrive like a plant in the field"* (v. 6-7a). As the child, Israel, grew, Ezekiel records that God continued to pay attention to her: *" . . . you grew, matured, and became very beautiful. Your breasts were formed, your hair grew, but you were naked and bare" (v7b).* This is extraordinarily personal, and sexually descriptive language.

"When I passed by you again and looked upon you, indeed your time was the time of love; so I spread My wing over you and covered your nakedness. Yes, I swore an oath to you and entered into a covenant with you, and you became Mine," says the Lord God." (V.8)

The passage goes on to explain the efforts God, as an interested, caring Husband, made to tenderly, royally, lavishly adorn Israel, with expensive fabrics and jewelry, with gold and silver, and fine perfumes. He even fed her special delicacies and anointed her with costly oils.

But what did she do with the gifts He enhanced her beauty with? She spent them to attract other lovers! Note, in the following description of her marital unfaithfulness, the overlay of descriptions of being spiritually unfaithful:

" 'But you trusted in your own beauty, played the harlot because of your fame, and poured out your harlotry on everyone passing by who would have it. You took some of your garments and adorned multicolored high places (places for idol worship) for yourself, and played the harlot on them. Such things should not happen, nor be. You have also taken your beautiful jewelry from My gold and My silver, which I had given you, and made for yourself male images (idols) and played the harlot with them. You took your embroidered garments and covered them, and you set My oil and My incense before them. Also My food which I gave you—the pastry of fine flour, oil, and honey which I fed you—you set it before them as sweet incense; and so it was,' says the Lord God." (V.15-19)

God is describing Israel's act of turning away from worshipping and loving Him only and turning instead to interact with the gods of the nations, even making images (idols for worship) out of the gold and silver God had provided her with out of His affection for her.

Ezekiel 23 has an even more graphic explanation of how the romance between God and unfaithful Israel felt to Him. The following is a description of Jerusalem's political and religious unfaithfulness to the God who had forever chosen her as the place for His dwelling; again, it is important to note the types of words used in this description, as they touch on lust and even pornography:

" . . . she (Jerusalem) carried her prostitution still further. She saw men portrayed on a wall, figures of Chaldeans portrayed in red, ***15*** *with belts around their waists and flowing turbans on their heads; all of them looked like Babylonian chariot officers, natives of Chaldea.* ***16*** *As soon as she saw them, she lusted after them and sent messengers to them in Chaldea.* ***17*** *Then the Babylonians came to her, to the bed of love, and in their lust they defiled her . . .* ***18*** *When she carried on her prostitution openly and exposed her naked body, I turned away from her in disgust, just as I had turned away from her sister.* ***19*** *Yet she became more and more promiscuous as she recalled the days of her youth, when she was a prostitute in Egypt.* ***20*** *There she lusted after her lovers, whose genitals were like those of donkeys and whose emission was like that of horses.* ***21*** *So you longed for the lewdness*

of your youth, when in Egypt your bosom was caressed and your young breasts fondled." (NIV)

The Idolatry/Adultery connection

Wow!! If you listen closely you can hear the tremendous pain in the heart of God, the perfect Lover, who had held nothing back in the offer of His love, protection, and lavish provision to Israel, the object of His affection in this story. Nevertheless, there came a day when, broken-hearted, He said to Israel: *"You are an adulterous wife, who takes strangers instead of her husband."* (Ezekiel 16:32)

I could spend the rest of this book unpacking the topic, but allow me instead to cut to the chase and share the insight that I was sensing from my Holy Teacher:

A) Once you start to look into scripture for references to the sacred relationship that God wanted to establish with Israel (and, seeing Israel as an example, with all humanity), you soon stumble into foundational descriptive references to His relational design and desire for interaction with humanity as being *like to one of marriage;*

B) Once you start tracking Israel's history of her "marriage" to God, you soon stumble into references to her repeatedly sliding into unfaithfulness to her "husband", marital unfaithfulness that is characterized in many texts by idolatry—that is, the worship of the (false) gods of other nations.

C) Once you start to track those sad chapters of Israel's history, you find the writers of the sacred text often accusing Israel not only of idolatry, but of adultery.

In short, I find that there is a peculiar, interactive relationship in the biblical texts between the concept of adultery and idolatry: to God, apparently *adultery* feels like *idolatry*, and *idolatry* feels like and is equal to *adultery*. God saw Israel's repetitive decision to turn away from the pure worship and love of her Redeemer/Husband and to enter into idolatry in some real way as a choice to enter into union with someone else, that is, as a choice by Israel to commit adultery.

When Israel turned away from God to idols, she was saying, "God, whatever it is you offer me, it is not enough." She was stating that regardless of what the writer of Psalm 23 had said, in spite of the fact that the Lord is her shepherd, *she is still in want; she is going to be defined by need*. And so she will turn to another for her needs to be met.

According to scripture, over and over again, that turning brought significant pain to God. And the pain brought distance: Isaiah 59:1-2 says: *"Behold, the Lord's hand is not shortened, that it cannot save; nor His ear heavy, that it cannot hear. But your iniquities have separated you from your God; and your sins have hidden His face from you, so that He will not hear."*

The fallout of choosing porn

As I was standing there in Nairobi between two towering displays of pornography, God's whisper reached my spirit with this impression: "When you willfully say 'yes' to the false intimacy that pornography offers, you are saying 'no' to the intimate union I offer; you are saying that what I provide is not enough. You are, in that action, choosing not just to turn to the adultery of sex outside of sacred marriage; you are choosing spiritual adultery, choosing to bow to an idol, to worship another god, to serve another provider, in fact you are choosing *to have union with a different supernatural entity.*

"Furthermore, that action of turning away from Me, or rejecting My capacity as your sole provider, will have ramifications that extend far beyond your own self: it will eventually require Me to agree with your choice, to allow you to have what you want, and to distance Myself from you, and this will invite, in place of My presence, a curse to visit you. I respond to your pure love with a blessing that extends to a thousand generations; but if you choose to turn deliberately from such love, this will not only bring pain to you, and to Me, but also will bring sadness— literally, a curse— to three or four generations of your family. Although such is difficult to comprehend, you must trust Me, understand, and believe this to be true.

"Beyond your choice to turn away from Me—from Truth, from Light, from Perfect Love, and all that is Good— you are choosing to have intercourse, deeper than you are at all aware of, with Darkness. Choosing pornographic intimacy is not a simple matter of you, all by yourself, interacting in isolation with random, two-dimensional naked women; your choice of pornographic intercourse is you literally choosing to make love with the kingdom of Darkness."

Unplugging porn's power

Last night, from our apartment in Israel, I was interacting rather aggressively (in a sacred sense) with a dear Pastor in his late 50's who is struggling to walk in purity. As we wrote back and forth, wrestling for his freedom, he texted at one point that he appreciated my tenacity.

I had to stop for a moment and figure out why it is that I am tenacious about this battle. I am sure there are many reasons, and I won't elaborate on them all here. But one in particular came rushing to the forefront of my thoughts and I'll share it with you now: I am tenacious about this whole purity and pornography battle because I am sick of being scammed, sick of being lied to, sick and tired of being taken. And I hate to hear that my brothers are similarly being sold the same lie I was peddled, and that as a result my sisters around the world are suffering intensely as the men in their lives are entangled in profound compromise. Although I may be a truly liberated poster-child for God's Mercy and Grace, I also have tremendous regrets: I lost at least 15 years of my life to the lie of what pornography pretended to offer. I hate that I was so stupid, so simple, so gullible. I was too long the fool written of in the book of Proverbs. Once the Holy Creator of heaven and earth invaded my space with the truth that pornography was a means whereby I was being (to some degree, literally) screwed by the devil, the *DECEPTION* that had been energizing my pornographic intercourse was removed, and I found myself being offered my own will back, by Jesus' own pierced hands. With that offering, the opportunity for me to say "NO" became an eventual, lasting reality.

The devil is a liar. And I hate the fact that for *so long I had been in bed with a liar.* I am tenacious in my work with men now because I want to offer them the same awakening that God brought to me, and to see the lies in their own minds unplugged, their own abused wills and sexuality returned to them, and their freedom stepped into and sustained by the Truth that sets us free.

The reader will recall that I am only writing this book in an attempt to help see you walk in absolute freedom as well. And before we go any further, I want to make sure you don't wait any longer to take up the invitation into clarity and wholeness that has perhaps been evading you for a long time. I want to make the most of our time together right now. For embedded within these first few pages of this book may be the very keys of revelation you need to finally, truthfully start to take stock of your own situation and make a new choice to untangle yourself from the devastation and dominion of untruth.

Wake up call: taking the bull by the horns

If you, dear reader, are someone who has been wrestling desperately with the terrible cycle of repeated interaction with pornographic intimacy, please know that freedom from the dominion of pornography is directly tied to the end of any deception in our hearts and minds in reference to pornography's deeply personal spiritual agenda. So as a means of Holy War, I want to close this chapter with a call to courageous clarity, and clarified courage. The following are statements of aggressive truth that I want to invite you to read through and ponder deeply. When you are ready to make them your own, with the Holy Spirit's help, please read through them again as a declaration over your life and choices.

From now on, I recognize that I simply cannot "have my cake and eat it too" any longer—- I cannot live as if I can have both an ongoing affair with darkness AND an ongoing personal relationship with Holy God.

I understand now from looking at the truth of the scriptures in this chapter that if I am going to continue to willfully engage in pornographic intimacy, I will do so knowing that, to God, my actions will feel like rejection—even an expression of hatred toward Him.

From now on, I realize that if I am going to continue to willfully engage in pornographic intimacy, my actions will at some point require God to distance Himself from me, even inviting Him, according to scripture, to visit three to four generations of my family with the negative results of such separation because of my choices.

From now on, I realize that if I am going to continue to willfully engage in pornographic intimacy, I understand that I will do so thinking only of myself and the meeting of my own primal needs. There can be no two ways about it: I realize now that if I still want to pursue pornographic intimacy, I must admit that I do not care primarily about God, my wife (or future wife, if I am

single), my children, or my children's children, or even their children beyond them. Instead, by my choice to continue to pursue pornographic intimacy, I understand that I would be deliberately trading our collective well-being, as I run over anyone in an effort to primarily value and meet my own needs.

Furthermore, from now on, I understand that if I am going to willfully engage in pornographic intimacy, I will do so knowing that, although I have prayed "the sinners' prayer" and have identified myself as a "Christian" , I am in fact NOT really a lover of God, am NOT really a Christ-follower, NOT really a disciple, but am, by God's definition, an idolater.

Dear reader, with the aid of the sword of scriptural truth cutting away all deception from our thinking, please ask yourself: "Are the above conclusions really what I want?" I think it is high time for us to man-up to what's really been going on in our private worlds. There must be no more deception in your thoughts or actions—from this point on, understand that ***if you choose to continue willfully pursuing pornographic intimacy, you will not be sinning in ignorance any longer.***

Perhaps when it is presented with such clarity, the healthy choice is easy to make. Perhaps you would say in your heart, "I know at the core that I really don't want to express anything *close* to hatred toward God, nor do I want to hurt my family in any way, or to be identified as an idolator. I now can see that I HAVE TO CHOOSE which lover will be mine. I cannot serve two masters any longer."

After a time of reflection, if you feel ready to move toward lasting change, I invite you to pray the following prayer:

With the help of the Holy Spirit, I acknowledge my profound level of deception, and my profound error in repeatedly, willfully surrendering to pornography. I hereby renounce my affair with pornographic intimacy for the sin that it is. I cry out to You, God Most High, to truly save me and forgive my courtship with such deep deception. I now ask for and embrace the proper Fear of the Lord, which is the beginning of wisdom and the end of folly. May the blood of Christ and the Holy Spirit of God help me as I earnestly, aggressively, honestly pursue a more complete understanding of true repentance. Prepare my heart now for the transcendent beauty and consecration of Holy Romance with Jesus Christ, the Lover of my soul. Amen.

Chapter 3 Courting Insanity

Driving down I-90 near Spokane a few years ago, I flipped on the FM radio in my '87 Chevy C10 pickup and caught a Christian talk-show, mid-program. Immediately riveted to the topic, I was stunned as I heard the radio preacher broadcast something to this effect: "Now there is no hocus-pocus going on behind pornography; it's just a bad habit, plain and simple. It has no power of its own. You don't need to be afraid of it—if you're involved in it, you just need to stop. Just say 'no' to it."

Wow—wouldn't it have been nice for me if all I had to do was say "no" to porn? That could have saved me more than a decade of insanity. My immediate thought on hearing this speaker was to think, first of all, "He has no idea what he is talking about!" And the second thought I had was that, although I have never met the man, I could tell you that he has never personally been under the addictive power of pornography. Porn—powerless? A simple bad habit— like chewing with your mouth open, or forgetting to put the lid down on the toilet after taking a leak? You've got to be kidding!

On the road again in Idaho only a few weeks later, I happened to catch another radio preacher, again speaking to his audience about pornography. This time the message sounded like this: "Interacting with Pornography is like drinking from a cup full of coffee grounds and cigarette ashes—its disgusting and horrible tasting; if you're considering drinking from that cup, just walk away, knowing that *it has nothing appealing to offer you.*"

Again I was stunned by this well-intentioned but grossly ignorant advice: the speaker was honestly suggesting that not only was porn powerless, but it actually had no appeal! For a second time, I knew there was no way that the voice of Christian leadership that I was hearing on the radio had any personal experience with the supernatural cocktail I'd encountered in the form of pornography.

As this book unfolds through the following chapters, I hope to help you contemplate the very serious question of *what is really going on behind the scenes in pornographic intercourse*; I want us to better understand the question: *Why does pornography work?*, that is, *Why and how does it seem to successfully enslave so many people?* In so doing I hope to also explore a related question: *How is it that so many in Christians circles—even among leaders in Christian circles—are clueless about it, clueless about providing truly lasting, effective help for the many who want out of its clutches?*

A look at the facts

To give a more realistic picture of the power and extent of porn than I heard on my truck radio, let's look at the statistics recorded primarily by the Barna Group and Covenant Eyes, reported in an article entitled, 15 Mind-Blowing Statistics About Pornography And The Church, by Luke Gibbons:

1. Over 40 million Americans are regular visitors to porn sites. The average visit lasts 6 minutes and 29 seconds
2. There are around 42 million porn websites, which totals around 370 million pages of porn.
3. The porn industry's annual revenue is more than the NFL, NBA, and MLB combined. It is also more than the combined revenues of ABC, CBS, and NBC.
4. 47% of families in the United States reported that pornography is a problem in their home.
5. Pornography use increases the marital infidelity rate by more than 300%.
6. Eleven is the average age that a child is first exposed to porn, and 94% of children will see porn by the age of 14.

7. 56% of American divorces involve one party having an "obsessive interest" in pornographic websites.
8. 70% of Christian youth pastors report that they have had at least one teen come to them for help in dealing with pornography in the past 12 months.
9. 68% of church-going men and over 50% of pastors view porn *on a regular basis*. Of young Christian adults 18-24 years old, 76% actively search for porn.
10. 59% of pastors said that married men seek their help for porn use.
11. 33% of women aged 25-and-under search for porn at least once per month.
12. Only 13% of self identified Christian women say they have never watched porn – 87% of Christian women say they have.
13. 55% of married men and 25% of married women say they watch porn at least once a month.
14. 57% of pastors say porn addiction is the most damaging issue in their congregation. And 69% say porn has adversely impacted the church.
15. Only 7% of pastors say their church has a program to help people struggling with pornography

Pretty impressive stats for a topic that my Christian radio told me "has no hocus-pocus empowering it", and that basically "has no appeal" to the common man.

Beyond these statistics, here's what I know from personal experience: engaging with pornography is like experimenting with powerfully addictive hallucinogenic drugs. Seriously.

This is your brain, on porn

If you are not yet aware of that well-documented scientific reality, please take the time to look into it. You do not have to look long online to find immediate answers to the question, "Are there similarities between pornography and drug addiction?" (for example, see article here: fightthenewdrug.org How Porn Affects The Brain Like A Drug).

It's pretty common knowledge that from the first experience an individual has with some drugs, one runs the danger of being so impacted physically, deep inside the chemical sensory administration center of the brain, that a powerful physical and psychological compulsion is often developed—even in that very first interaction—a compulsion to unlock and repeat the same extraordinary brain chemistry sensation. Science has discovered that the same type of deep mental interaction and ground-laying activity for compulsion takes place in the pornographic intercourse experience. In fact, the reality is so deep and physical that it makes visible, physical changes in the landscape of your actual brain!

I'm not going to spend too much time trying to prove this to you; even many secular writers are making statements that should be a huge wake up call to us that there is much more than meets the eye regarding porn. (For more on this topic, see the following articles in secular media: July 11, 2017 article by Peter Hess, entitled, This is Your Brain on Porn, published on inverse.com; June 2, 2011 article by Naomi Wolf, entitled, Is Pornography Driving Men Crazy?, published by Project Syndicate; 9 May, 2017 article by Simon Copland, entitled, The Many Reasons People are Having Less Sex, published on bbc.com).

From my end, I am trying to say loudly and clearly to any reader who is entangled with porn: You cannot engage in pornography casually, and not have it affect you. You must wake up to the reality: *the pornographic intercourse you are engaging in is altering you, damaging you, killing you.* In my opinion, porn is a long, drawn out form of suicide.

What does it look like in real life? Insanity. For me, pornography led me into a slow rise of insanity.

The view from my room

I'll never forget the first time I bought a pornographic magazine as a married man. The year was 1984. My wife and I had just moved to a new town where she had taken a job as an elementary teacher. Her career was just beginning. She was fresh out of college. We were in our first months of marriage. Unschooled (I had to leave higher education due to lack of finances), I had to find work and did my best to do so, eventually landing a solid job in construction. But before that opened up, I found myself with time on my hands, and ended up one afternoon at a small-town used bookstore, as I have always loved to read. Browsing around innocently, I unexpectedly came across a stock of second-hand Playboys. $1 each. As my heart rate soared with the wild challenge this offer posed to me, impulsively, I bought one. I sold my conscience that day for a buck.

Dear reader, stop for a moment and tell yourself this truth: *no matter how small the initial price tag, you can never afford the cost of pornography*. And even if its only $1 that you are spending on it, when the cost is taken from a budget that is supposed to be for your wife and you to live on, it is stealing. In this (and in a thousand other very significant ways), ***pornography always involves dishonesty and always includes stealing.***

Driven by towering curiosity and the lure of a cheap, exotic high adventure, I paid $1, took home one magazine, and found myself delighted with what I'd purchased: here were photos of women who looked me directly in the eye, smiled, and invited me into the wonder of their beauty. Best of all, there were apparently no strings attached: in order for them to share with me all they had, no efforts were demanded on my part to do the work of developing healthy relationship. Unlike the work I was finding a good marriage required to open the doors to a sacred woman's heart and soul, the $1 offer of pornographic intercourse really required no effort, and demanded no relational courage from me. It appeared that the smiling women in that $1 mag offered, via their poses and the connection of my own self-stimulation, free, unfettered sex, the answer to my unspoken dreams. I did not hesitate; I took their bait.

It would be a long time before I came to see it, but in case you have little experience with this reality, let me point it out right here: ***Pornographic sex is tremendously cowardly; it is tied directly to indolence, laziness, slothfulness, idleness. If you wish to be well, these character flaws, too, must be acknowledged and renounced, and with the help of the Holy Spirit, replaced with the sacred courage and initiative that healthy relationships must require.***

Diving deeper into the fantasy I'd spread before my eyes that day, masturbation brought a sensational, explosive end to my adventure, and then immediately plunged me into the horrible, nearly overwhelming reality of my sin. As much as I had just been stunned by the beauty on display, I was now left with astonishing horror, guilt, and shame.

Quickly confessing my error to God and then declaring I would NEVER do that again, I ran outside, horrified, and threw the magazine into the dumpster outside our apartment building.

Phew! That was that! Thank God for 1 John 1:9, right? Confess it and its dealt with!! Walk away from that prayer with a clean slate! That afternoon, I turned my back on my momentary lapse in character and walked away, thinking all was well. (Obviously I had a lot to learn about what REAL confession is; but that would come another year . . .)

Dumpster diving

The next day, while my noble wife was at work at the Christian school where she was a first grade teacher, I was halfway through the morning when I found myself rushing outside and *climbing into* the dumpster, sifting through piles of stinking trash, until I found the magazine I had tossed the day before. I then brought it back into our apartment and again interacted with it, re-experiencing the rise of transcendent fascination, delight, and wonder of sexual stimulation in the face of such easy, all-encompassing acceptance that these smiling nudes seemed to offer me; my heart physically hammered with the adventure, and then again, as soon as climax was achieved, I experienced the immediate plummeting crash of reality, self-loathing, shame, and deep panic about what I had done. Then the magazine was again relegated to the dumpster. Confession again was made a second time, perhaps with more effort, more seriousness. A new commitment to stoic integrity was announced to myself.

Still, the next day, again I fled to the dumpster, hoping for round three; but to my dismay, it had been emptied. The compulsion in my mind would go unsatiated.

This particular experience— that first porn magazine I purchased as an adult and my attempts to get rid of it in that dumpster—took place in late 1984. Although pornographic intercourse became a sin I would engage in many times over the next ten years, to the best of my knowledge I never repeated that dumpster diving aspect of the interaction. But still to this day, 35 years later, I react physically whenever I walk past a dumpster; part of my physical brain has registered a permanent link between dumpsters and the release of the high adventure, pleasure neurotransmitter that exploded in my mind only once, way back in 1984. That's a glimpse into the tremendous power hiding behind pornographic intercourse. And that's insane.

I don't know where you're at in your journey, but if you are repeatedly interacting with pornography as a part of your story, then again I want to see the Truth break through any lies that are sustaining your capacity to play around with pornographic intercourse as if it is all still under your control and nothing you are doing will end up having any lasting affect on you. You are being played by Darkness. Stop kidding yourself: *Attending to such a powerful drug as porn will drive you insane*.

Chapter 4 Fear at the Wheel

By the grace of God and the power of the blood of Jesus and by the deliberate sharing of the word of my own testimony, I have walked in freedom from the dominion of porn since 1999. Hallelujah—that is a miracle! Find, in my saying so, the good news you need to hear: ***Jesus Christ still sets prisoners free; He still does miracles***. That's not hype; it's truth. If you are in need of a miracle along these lines, please read on. As Zach Williams so triumphantly sings about Him: *"If you've got chains, He's a chain breaker!"*

They say "hindsight is 20/20 vision." Now that the years of darkness are behind me, I find it important for me to continue to look back and dissect as best as possible the role porn played in my life for fifteen plus years. I do so in an attempt to allow you to look through the valuable assist that Hindsight gives me today.

I could not have seen it at the time, but as pornographic intercourse became a part of my life for the first 13 years of my marriage, there were definite contributing factors that seemed to play into my entanglement with it. I want us to look for a moment at what some of those contributing factors were, in an effort to cut off similar cycles that you may find yourself involved in without knowing.

Scared to face the music

First off there was in my life at the time the contributing factor of my being seriously *afraid of the necessary pain associated with overcoming challenges and embracing the responsibilities of adulthood*. You would not have read it in my face, but internally I would do anything to avoid pain. At the time, I was afraid of many things, but one fear really was played on in a big way in the development of my connection to pornographic intercourse: that is, the fear of really facing challenges head on.

As a young, newly married college drop out, there were lots of enormous challenges on my horizon: economic challenges, occupational limitations, a deep lack of identity. Each of these dared me to overcome, dared me to rise up and take responsibility for myself and my household. It was all a part of normal entry into manhood and I should have been man enough to face and work through each of these challenges; but in truth, they scared me to death.

Of course my fear of facing challenges invited conflict into our home. When conflicts naturally came up between

Caryn Beth and I (as they would in any marriage) she kindly radiated the confidence needed to move ahead, whereas I backed quietly into a corner psychologically. At the mere hint of conflict between us, I felt embarrassed at my lack of leadership skills; self-defense was always my posture.

Looking back on it now, I can easily see that at the time I thought far too highly of myself. As it does to all young men, life was forcing me to look in the mirror and acknowledge that I had some gaping holes in my personal development, glaring lack that needed attention. Rather than facing the music and finding solutions to the challenges in front of me, I turned away: it all seemed like too much for me to face. I became depressed, withdrawn.

For better AND for worse

During this dark period, I would at times find myself engaged with pornography as a means of "therapy". Here's why: My own unredeemed introspection led to darkened thinking on how much my own rights had been trampled by life, how much I had been overlooked and undervalued by society itself, how much I really *deserved* to be worshipped and was not being worshipped, how much *I really needed and deserved to feel better*. Porn quietly offered a way to make me feel *better*. So went my thoughts on many an occasion.

At other times, as peers in our church community advanced in their careers and economic status, looking at the world through my dark glasses at my stagnant development left me feeling so BAD that I thought I might as well go and do something BAD, so that the shame I felt from being such a societal loser would fit properly. So porn would quietly offer to make me feel *worse*.

It's all so clearly insane to me now, and it is with a very heavy heart and tear-stained face that I reflect on this period. Again, I only share the sad trail of thoughts with you here in hopes of saving you from having to experience the hell I lived with silently for too long.

Tragically, during my first year of marriage, instead of embracing the invitation to learn and grow in the challenging arena of adulthood *with* Caryn Beth— the deeply beautiful, and bright, hopeful ally I'd promised to faithfully love— I retreated from the painful challenges life posed me and began to turn to a different partner: Pornographic Intercourse. It offered me a quick trip to a feel-better/feel worse place. During that first year of our marriage, I began to use porn to medicate, to help me escape, to hide me from pain.

I've said it earlier in this book but I'll say it again: In my simple mind, the naked women who silently offered themselves to me via porn gave me attention that felt genuine, felt like respect. It didn't matter that I hadn't earned it. It felt real. It felt (momentarily) great. And, devoid as it was of any prerequisite conversational skills, it was so easy to attain.

I now believe this false intimacy (that at times in my insanity even included me *talking* to the photos I was staring at) was in fact a form of self-worship, for me to so receive such apparent adoration of self in the secret recesses of my mind.

A special lake for cowards

Years later, I recall another breakthrough moment when the Holy Spirit helped me begin to honestly review the depth of depraved, warped thinking that I had been entertaining. He challenged me one day as I was reading through the book of Revelation with Him. I was in chapter 21 one morning when I came across these words in verses 6-8 that stopped me dead in my tracks:

"And He said to me, ". . . I will give of the fountain of the water of life freely to him who thirsts. {Wow, I thought: that could be me!! I am so thirsty for that . . . } *He who overcomes shall inherit all things, and I will be his God and he shall be My son.* {Again I thought, wow—that could be me! How awesome!! } *But the cowardly, unbelieving, abominable, murderers, sexually immoral, sorcerers,*

idolaters, and all liars shall have their part in the lake which burns with fire and brimstone, which is the second death."

Cue up the scary soundtrack music; this was suddenly very, very serious:

My eyes were arrested by that phrase, *"But the cowardly . . ."*
"*Cowardly?* (I was conversing now with the Holy Spirit) *"Are you highlighting that word in reference to ME?!?!"*

"*Yes I am,"* came the very solemn reply from my Wonderful Counselor.

I did not understand; *"You think of ME as a coward?"* I asked, with no small amount of exasperation driving my question.

A quiet sigh from heaven; then: *"Yes, I do."*

Incredulous, as I thought back over how brave I considered myself to be, I voiced another question: *"How is that possible?"*

"When you look at your continued, willful pornographic involvement as your means of finding escape from things

that make you uncomfortable, you are choosing to remain childish; you must see that you really are acting like a coward."

Although I had never contemplated it before, immediately the truth of this statement hit me like a hammer, crushing the lie of legitimacy that pornography had been holding up in front of itself. In Nairobi, I had been completely surprised to consider that my interacting with pornography had been not only *adulterous*, but even *idolatrous*; now I was similarly shocked and profoundly concerned to find out that my cyclical intercourse with pornography was also identifying me with a serious level of *cowardice*; and not only cowardice on its own, as if that weren't bad enough—*this was a God-defined and identified cowardice that was directly connected in this verse with a one-way trip to a lake which burns with fire and brimstone*. That's pretty heavy.

As my adrenaline climbed with this contemplation, I read verse 8 again: *"But the cowardly, unbelieving, abominable, murderers, sexually immoral, sorcerers, idolaters, and all liars shall have their part in the lake which burns with fire and brimstone, which is the second death."*

With the sacred, faithfully wounding help of the Holy Spirit, my concern and appropriate conviction skyrocketed.

Reading, as I was now, with the help of His lamp to my feet, I could see that *cowardly* was not the only thing in this list that I needed to be concerned about being labeled with: Pornography, I felt the Spirit slowly, firmly impress upon my heart, was also connected with *unbelief* in me, with my being *abominable*, *sexually immoral (of course)*, *idolatrous (as we've already seen)*, and a *liar (ditto).* I was especially concerned about the *liar* label, as the verse clearly labeled as doomed not just *some* liars, but *ALL* liars. I did not feel the label of 'murderer' or 'sorcerer' necessarily fit me, but the rest of this verse had me suddenly very appropriately afraid of inheriting my part in the lake that burns . . .

Orchestrated fall from grace

Again, an impression: *"It is time for your struggle with fear to be unplugged, for your pain-avoidance to end, and actually for your fear-center to be appropriately rewired. It's time for you to stop being afraid of pain, and to start deliberately entering with confidence into responsibility for the normal, necessarily difficult challenges of life outside of Eden. You can do that, but you can't do that if you are afraid of the wrong things."*

This was a terribly unsettling consideration for me to entertain. Although I knew this was the Good Shepherd leading me to a far better place, for me, things had to get worse before they got better: I had to let go of my old coping mechanisms before I could find a better response to fear than the hollow offering of pornographic gratification. I did not know how to go about that. So I ignored the invitation to change, and in so doing unwittingly invited the Holy Spirit to draft for me a more drastic transformation.

What followed was that in an act of tremendous personal love, transcendent wisdom, and creativity, God very publicly orchestrated my sudden removal from ministry in Kenya, so that He could best melt me down and reprogram me. One equatorial sultry March afternoon, during a tremendously stressful week of overwork on my part, as the chief of security at our mission station I had to make a difficult arrest of an intruder; in the chaos of my trying to deal with the culprit, I lost my temper and (very uncharacteristically) slapped the (Kenyan) man across the face. Several school board meetings hastily followed on the heels of the episode, as the school involved was very concerned about the possibility of the story being reported in the news as a racial incident. For the protection of the school's interests and reputation, it was deemed by the school board that it would be best to remove me from ministry and have me leave Kenya immediately. Three days after the event, I sat alone on a KLM flight, weeping my way down the runway, flying away from life as I knew it. (Caryn Beth and our children followed me to the USA a month later.)

Although the abrupt, unforeseen end of our 5 years in Kenya was terribly embarrassing to me, in His mercy God pulled it off without overly shaming me, and did so without anyone knowing anything about the struggle with pornography that I was still dancing with. He brought an abrupt, decisive end to my work and forced me to rethink my whole life and world.

I do not think any such end to ministry would have ever taken place if I had not been at the same time also engaged in pornographic intercourse. I learned then, by that experience, the truth so clearly written in Galatians 6:7,8a: *"Do not be deceived, God is not mocked; for whatever a man sows, that he will also reap. For he who sows to his flesh will of the flesh reap corruption . . ."* Even while growing as a believer and engaged in kingdom of heaven work, I had also periodically been willfully, deliberately sowing to my flesh—investing in the well-being of my flesh, thinking all the while that it did not really matter and that mercy would continue to protect me from any negative repercussions; but God, because He cared so much about my well-being, in one sense allowed me to push His presence away from me, and in the vacuum of His presence, allowed the seeds I'd sown to bring about the destruction I'd invested in.

The experience was tremendously and necessarily humiliating and almost broke my mind entirely. A full year of PTSD anxiety followed, eventually landing me in the hospital and lining me up for months of counseling. That terrible/wonderful story of my redemption would take up too many pages here. But suffice it to say, God was going to make sure that if I wanted to be His son, He wanted me to be done with inappropriate fear, done with avoiding pain, done with self-soothing and escape.

What's the worst that could happen?

I remember one sleepless night, months after our return to life and blue-collar work in the States. By now I was wrestling with clinical levels of fear, awake one night trying to ignore the piercing physical pain that acute anxiety was manifesting in my left side. I finally broke the silence with a desperate prayer, thinking of my own experience as if being in a small boat, at sea amidst a great tempest: *"Jesus, won't you please take me out of this storm?!!"* I cried out.

The night around me was silent in reply. I continued, *"Won't you please calm the wind and stop these terrible waves?"*

In my heart I felt a very clear impression, that same still, small holy voice, whispering to me in reply:

"I will not stop the storm, but I will teach you to sleep through it."

"WHAT?!" I shouted back!

The Whisper continued: "What is the worst that can happen to you?"

I knew the answer to that—my heart immediately shouted back into the night: *"I could lose my mind!"*

"No, that is not the worst that could happen to you."

I tried to defend my position. *"Well, if I lost my mind, I would lose my job. We would lose our home! I could lose our children! I could lose my wife!"* Horrible images of me holed up on a cot in a homeless shelter, entirely alone, flashed through my mind. Then came a picture of me locked up in a psychiatric ward of a hospital. Certainly, that was the worst that could happen to me, right?

I could tell the Voice was waiting for a better answer to His question. I paused, considering what fate might possibly be worse than losing my sanity altogether.

As my words failed, His voice began again: *"I want you to consider what it would be like to have your whole world turn against you— your wife, your children, your entire extended family, everyone you ever knew, anyone you might ever meet—all turned against you. Imagine that, and then know this—as long as you still had Me, you could endure that. The loss of all human support is not the worst that could happen to you."*

I was astonished by these words. Yet there was a clear sense of unshakeable truth behind them.

"And not only all of humanity— imagine all of Hell gathered against you as well, the entire force of evil throughout the universe. Imagine it! Everything other than Me that exists—turned against you! Even THAT would not be the worst that could happen to you. Even if you faced that—if you still had Me on your side, you could make it through."

After a brief pause, allowing me to contemplate this staggering idea, the whisper continued.

"The worst that could happen to you is that I could leave you. I could abandon you. I could leave you alone.

"That you could not ever endure. That alone is something for you to consider fearing."

Another quiet pause ensued before the voice continued, soft and steady.

"This fear, the single-most legitimate reason for you to be afraid, this you will never have to face. Hear me now: this will never happen to you, for I love you. I love you with an everlasting love. I have decided to love you. You are mine and I am yours. Nothing will ever be able to separate you from My love.

"Believe what I am telling you. You are fearful. You feel afraid. The enemy has tried to make you believe that you a coward. You feel like you need to protect yourself from pain, and so you create illegitimate places of escape from imagined danger. But you were made to face pain, not to fear it! You were made for courage, not for cowardice! I want to help you become brave! You must learn what it means to be a real man; and, if necessary, you must learn to sleep through a storm."

Walking decisively away from the dominion of pornography in my life meant that I had to admit to a level of cowardice that had to be identified and deliberately uprooted, divorced from my existence and identity, and replaced with the boldness that comes from knowing that no matter what difficulties I might face in life, I would face them knowing the all-powerful, perfect love of God was my unshakable anchor, my unalterable reality.

Here's the bottom line for me now: in the face of imagined fears, I thought I needed to feel good; I thought I needed to be afraid of pain, afraid of anything that might make me lose track of feeling okay. Now I know that is a lie! Now I know that I'm going to be okay, even if, for one reason or other, I don't *feel* okay.

Biblically, the lie-breaking, power-infused truth sounds like this:

The Lord is my shepherd; therefore, I shall no longer be defined by need. I will no longer let need push me off balance, and into the darkness. The Lord is my shepherd; even though at times I must walk close to things that would naturally make me afraid, I will fear no evil, because You, God, are FOREVER, INSEPARABLY with me.

Lamentations chapter 3:54-58 puts it this way:

"The waters flowed over my head;
I said, 'I am cut off!'
I called on Your name, O Lord,
From the lowest pit.
You have heard my voice:

'Do not hide Your ear from my sighing,
from my cry for help.'
You drew near on the day I called on You,
And said, 'Do not fear!'
O Lord, You have pleaded the case for my soul;
You have redeemed my life."

Chapter 5 Shots across my bow

"Jerusalem has sinned gravely,
Therefore she has become vile.
She did not consider her destiny;
Therefore her collapse was awesome . . ."
(from Lamentations 1)

1998

I think it was a vision, or maybe a dream. I don't remember now which it was. But I'll never forget the content broadcast across the screen in my mind, branding my wild soul with an ominous message.

In the vision/dream I could see the iron rails and timbers of a train track, long and serpentine, passing through rolling plains, under a scorching sun, unimaginably far out beyond all civilization to where the tracks finally came to a sudden and abrupt end. Just beyond the final section of track, I saw myself, alone, sitting cross legged and naked, wet with my own fluids. Beside me sat a stack of playboy magazines.

This would be my end, the vision explained to me with certainty, emotionless and stark as the Sahara. *I would get what I wanted: endless, uninhibited ecstasy* (and with it, absolute isolation, separation from everything other than the deadly sickness I was fondling).

I was tremendously shocked and appalled at the possibility the vision proposed; because God loved me desperately, His Spirit was again warning me, calling me to make a final break with pornographic intercourse, before the mess I was making of me became permanent.

"Lead me not into temptation." So reads a key part of the famous prayer Jesus taught His core students. In the original language, one scholar (whose work I have sadly been unable to track down in the years since I first read it) stated that embedded in the cultural context, being "led into temptation" had implicit in it the idea of taking a small one-man boat and rowing in it so far out to sea that the return to shore or the hope of rescue would never be even remotely possible. Such is the hidden end of addictive sin. Such is the fine print on the back of the contract of pornographic intercourse.

What life without God might feel like

God has clearly, openly decided to direct His kindness and love toward us; when we make friends with the enemy of all that is good for us, I sincerely suspect that there is an adjustment bureau in heaven that assigns angels to our case, releasing incident-based revelation to get our attention and bring us back from our slow rush to destroy our own lives. Such is my story: for once the Counselor started invading my double life with His truth and shepherding rod, He also released circumstances that helped with His efforts to awaken me to the danger of my poor choices. It was as if He was arranging things in my world in order to make sure I got this message: "Your sins are forcing me to distance myself from you, for your own good. If, by your repeatedly, willfully choosing dark intimacy, you really want to distance yourself from me, that can be arranged; I can work with that idea, and still honor your free will. So for the next few months, I am going to allow you to experience on a small scale what life without Me might feel like." There was tremendous wisdom and tenderest perfect love behind that revelation.

1998 and '99 was the timeframe of that celestially orchestrated experiment, and my final battle with duplicity, gross immaturity, and the dominion of darkness in my private world. The shocking expulsion from life in Kenya was a stunning wake-up for me, as for the first time I considered that my pet, secret errors might in fact have a serious negative impact in the real world. But as huge an event as my having been kicked out of international ministry was and the attending unofficial deporting from a country, it was not by any means the only circumstance I feel heaven's severe mercy orchestrated in my final transformation. There were several other uncanny events that took place in the span of only a few months, intense and unexplainably coincidental events that I am sure now were given to me to make sure I did not waste the monumental efforts of Jesus to enforce my deliverance, events sent to make sure I did not spurn the grace that my life to this point had been hedged in with, to make sure I came to the place where the appropriate, healthy fear of God became a prominent, constant companion of mine for the remainder of my life. I will share here just one of those strange occurrences.

As you read, if you are still deliberately making room for pornographic intimacy, know this: You need to be afraid. If you are still persisting in your duplicity, BE AFRAID, for something like what happened to me could very well be on your horizon. Get sober about this, and make the necessary effort to understand and fully believe this statement: *"Because of the Lord's great love, we are not consumed, because His compassions never fail."* (Lamentations 3:22) Another translator wrote it this way: *"We are still alive because the Lord's faithful love never ends!"* (ERV)

After the tremendous disgrace of my being expelled from our five years of life and ministry in Kenya, God was very kind in helping me find employment back in the United

States. As my wife diligently cleaned houses so that we could put our children back into private school, my putting in fifty plus hours a week of manual labor at a factory made room for us to be able to pay rent and keep clothes on our backs and food in our fridge. But as I mentioned in the previous chapter, at this point my mind was melting down with PTSD—after having destroyed our future in Kenya with my own hands, the stunning and embarrassing exit from Africa had left me deeply distrustful of both myself and my fellow man.

In the presence of such panic, even though I was aware that God was really pursuing me in a way I had never before experienced, I was still haunted with temptation to intimacy with lesser gods, constantly aware of their old offer of (false) refuge, and was mentally considering a momentary proverbial return to the very things I had previously vomited out of my life.

One Michigan evening, I pulled the beautiful, like-new-condition Chrysler New Yorker (my father in law had graciously given us) into the parking lot of the local video rental store, and went in, surfing for garbage. With the whole Kenyan incident having freaked me out, I now was too afraid to risk actually renting an "adult" video, but thought I might get away with just walking through the adult section of the huge store and seeing what I could feed my eyes with from the boxed videos on display.

I did not stay long, as I recall; I was not very comfortable in what I was doing. Still, I am sure I saw a lot of what should not be seen, consuming with my hungry eyes images that even on the covers of the videos were far from healthy. Then without checking out any videos, I returned to my waiting car.

Sliding into the tufted burgundy leather driver's seat of the New Yorker, I pulled the keys from my pocket and put them into the ignition. Like I had done every time I started a car since I had learned to drive at age 17, I then attempted to twist the ignition tumbler, expecting it to turn and the engine to burst into life. But the key would not turn. Over and over I tried, pulling the key out and reinserting it into the mechanism, making sure that in the nervous state I was in, having just walked out of a dark place mentally, I was not inadvertently forcing anything. But no matter what I tried, the key would not turn; the ignition could receive no signal to start the engine. Exasperated, I must have tried for 15 minutes to turn that key, but to no avail. I was marooned.

"How odd," I remember thinking; *"I wonder if it has anything to do with what I had just been doing?"* (Ya think?!? I still had tremendous levels of unbelief infecting my mind.)

Perplexed, I walked in the dark the three or four city blocks that night to our home. I left the car parked where it was until morning, and then made some phone calls and had it towed to a very professional high-end auto repair shop nearby. The mechanics dug into it and ordered the new ignition parts, telling me it would be a couple days before the part arrived and had been installed. The price would be a challenge for me to attend to on our limited budget, but at least the car would be back on the road.

I was relieved. Although the experience had been quite unsettling, it appeared I had dodged a bullet. I quickly concluded that there had been no connection between my looking at adult videos and the sudden arrest of my car. But apparently Heaven was not comfortable with that conclusion on my part and wanted to make sure I got the message that my dabbling with darkness had to come to a final end. So while I slept that night, another shot was fired across my bow.

This is your car, on porn. Any questions?

The next morning I got a call from the automotive repair shop owner. He was very apologetic as he explained to me that during the night, someone had jumped the fence and gone through his establishment, and had selected my car out of the many in his lot. He explained that someone had broken into my car and removed the whole dashboard, and then stolen the entire computer control module that was the brain of the vehicle. Now the ignition of the car was not the only thing missing; *its entire capacity to think had been taken away.* Now there was not just a small price to pay for the repairs; there was a two-thousand-plus dollar repair tag left in the wake of the intruder.

I was stunned.

And I deserved to have been stunned.

This incident was one of the last straws for me as I was being so powerfully courted by both Heaven and Hell, and was *still* trying to figure out how to have my proverbial cake and eat it too. The message was clear that I could NOT!

God was not afraid to spend my money, or disrupt my schedule, or give me enough rope to get myself into trouble. He is in fact not afraid to risk any and everything that can be shaken in an attempt to get us to value only that which is of lasting, unshakable value. He it is who kindly places before us life and death and says to us, with a passionate tremble in His voice: *Please choose life and not death!*

There is a sin that leads to death (see 1 John 5). I'm not sure Western Christianity really holds to that truth anymore, at least not in practice. I know that for a long time, I did not; but Jehovah does. And so He intervenes in the lives of those who stray from the life He has placed before them. In these (and several other similarly extraordinary and supernaturally orchestrated experiences) God was helping me find a way into the necessary confines of humility and its role in repentance.

Reading just this week through the book of Lamentations, I was moved by the following words in chapter 3 and their echoing description of my life in 1999:

"17 You have moved my soul far from peace;
I have forgotten prosperity.
18 And I said, 'My strength and my hope
Have perished from the Lord.'

"25 The Lord is good to those who wait for Him,
To the soul who seeks Him.
26 It is good that one should hope and wait quietly
For the salvation of the Lord.
27 It is good for a man to bear
The yoke in his youth.

"28 Let him sit alone and keep silent,
Because God has laid it on him;
29 Let him put his mouth in the dust—

There may yet be hope.
30 Let him give his cheek to the one who strikes him,
And be full of reproach.
31 For the Lord will not cast off forever.
32 Though He causes grief, yet He will show compassion
According to the multitude of His mercies.
33 For He does not afflict willingly,
Nor grieve the children of men."
From Lamentations 3

Along this vein, lest we think the above is only a description of the God of the Old Testament, please contemplate these life giving, tender words from Hebrews 12 as well:

" . . . consider (Jesus) who endured such hostility from sinners against Himself, lest you become weary and discouraged in your souls. You have not yet resisted to bloodshed, striving against sin. And you have forgotten the exhortation which speaks to you as to sons: 'My son, do not despise the chastening of the Lord, nor be discouraged when you are rebuked by Him; for whom the Lord loves He chastens, and scourges every son whom He receives.' If you endure chastening, God deals with you as with sons; for what son is there whom a father does not chasten? But if you are without chastening, of which all

have become partakers, then you are illegitimate and not sons. Furthermore, we have had human fathers who corrected us, and we paid them respect. Shall we not much more readily be in subjection to the Father of spirits and live?" (Hebrews 12: 3-9)

Chapter 6 Eyes and Hands

When I nervously picked up the New Yorker after it had finally been repaired, I admit that I was feeling a bit hemmed in by God. At the same time, sensing that the hedge around me might be a *good* thing, I began to ask some questions to the Spirit of God that was sharing the house of me: "Why are You three so adamant about this issue in my life? Why so serious about this sin? What is the big deal after all?" These were the puzzles I would carry around with me and mentally turn over and over like a Rubik's cube for a long time. But once I started asking them, powerful answers from scripture eventually started coming to my attention. I will share a few of them with you here.

God is adamant/insistent/unyielding about the severity of this sin because it is somehow different from other sins.

God is adamant about this sin because it invites darkness into union with us.

God is adamant about this sin because it forces not just us, but Him (by nature of His residing inside of us) into union with darkness. (Please see pages 150-155 for a fuller explanation of these claims.)

I believe it is with the prevention of these tragic dangers that Jesus augments for the listening crowds their understanding of the dangers of unrestrained lust, launching directly into a very important discussion of the dangers of pornographic intercourse.

"You have heard that it was said to those of old, You shall not commit adultery.' But I say to you that whoever looks at a woman to lust for her has already committed adultery with her in his heart. If your right eye causes you to sin, pluck it out and cast it from you; for it is more profitable for you that one of your members perish, than for your whole body to be cast into hell. And if your right hand causes you to sin, cut it off and cast it from you; for it is more profitable for you that one of your members perish, than for your whole body to be cast into hell."
(Matthew 5:27-30)

There is a lot going on in this text. Let me talk about a couple of key things God brought to my attention from this section of scripture during my awakening.

Guilty eyes

First off, Jesus is obviously making it clear that in His eyes, and for our sakes, there must be no mistake: *looking to lust after someone—that is, deliberately, illicitly staring (in a sexually objectifying manner and for the sake of purely selfish satisfaction of sexual hunger) at the physical beauty of someone— is not just similar to the sin of adultery: it IS the sin of adultery! Jesus doesn't care if I agree with His (re-)definition of "looking at a woman to lust." He is not asking the opinion or perspective of any of us on the issue. He is saying it straight up: this is how it is —lust in action, deliberately and unrestrainedly employed, is adultery! Period.*

Let's approach this in another way: if you happen to be one of the 68% of church-going men or the 50% of pastors who view porn on a regular basis, or if you are one of the 76% young Christian adults 18-24 years old, who actively search for porn, I would guess that within that staggering number, in spite of your undisciplined, wandering eyes, there are very few of you who have actually crossed the line and committed yourself to involvement in a "real" affair and have engaged in sexual intercourse, not just with a photo but with a "real" woman, one who is already married to someone else. Jesus approached *that* loophole we tend to hide behind—"Well, I may be struggling with a stronghold of LUST but at least

I'm not committing (nor ever would REALLY commit) adultery" loophole— and He says, "Nope: that defense doesn't stand in my court. ***When you willfully allow Lust to drive your actions, you are guilty of adultery. Case Closed!"*** *(Hear the gavel fall!)*

Let's stop here and consider the change that Jesus' simple redefinition of "Looking at a woman to lust" might have on your experience. Again, if you are one of the many still choosing to engage in pornographic intercourse, I bet your not having yet engaged in actual adultery has also been a deliberate choice of yours: you have not committed *actual* adultery, because in your mind it is on a whole new level of commitment to get involved in such an act. But if Jesus words of truth can hammer His standard into your mindset to such a degree that you will agree with Him and call pornographic intercourse what it really is—*real adultery*—then you will have a better handle on finally finding a way to say NO to porn's offer of false intimacy.

Here's what that looked like in practice for me: It was late in the year 1999 when a man at work broke away from a heated discussion taking place on down the production line we worked on and approached me abruptly. He knew very little about me other than that I had been in ministry in Kenya for 5 years. He had only one question to ask, and asked it bluntly: "Have you ever committed adultery?" the question totally blindsided me, as I had no relationship with this guy and sensed he had a low opinion of me already. But the Spirit of God was orchestrating a test for me: I could have said right away, "No—of course not!" In so stating, the self-righteous part of me would have made myself look good, might have made my character appear untarnished. But I sensed the Spirit of God standing there with me, inviting me to the healthy place that honesty would open, even if it came at the expense of my reputation. Had I ever committed adultery? I braced my shoulders and looked the man in the eyes, focusing on Jesus' redefinition of my engagement with porn: "Yes, I'm sorry to say, I have." It was all I said, all I felt allowed by the Holy Spirit to say at the moment. Immediately, the man turned and walked away, obviously disgusted. It was the first time I publicly owned up to the truth of my errors.

Before we go beyond this re-defining moment for me, let me throw another verse into the mix so we are fully aware of how God thinks about this. The writer of Hebrews 13:4 states emphatically: *"Marriage is honorable among all, and the bed undefiled; but fornicators and adulterers God will judge."* Hmmm. No ambiguity there! GOD WILL JUDGE FORNICATORS AND ADULTERERS! It's as if the two issues—fornication and adultery—are one and the same here in God's eyes. Maybe write that on a sticky note and adhere it to your mirror . . . Seriously!

Another foundational aspect of this discussion is that Matthew 5:32 makes it crystal clear that sexual immorality in marriage is the ONLY reason Jesus declared was legitimate grounds for divorce (divorce still being, as He states elsewhere, something He hates). *". . . I say to you that whoever divorces his wife for any reason except sexual immorality causes her to commit adultery; and whoever marries a woman who is divorced commits adultery."* That is a pivotal consideration for those who are willfully, cyclically, habitually entertaining the sexually immoral, adulterous activity that pornographic intercourse truly is. No two ways around it: you don't have to be a rocket scientist to understand from scripture that God does not overlook this erroneous pattern of living, nor does He encourage us to just be merciful and look the other way when it manifests in our relationships.

Higher ground: hard medicine

With these bright lights now illuminating my own shadows, I began to contemplate a course for healthy recovery from the pornographic infection I had been carrying for so long. In private conversation with the Wonderful Counselor, I eventually realigned and anchored my understanding to a new level of grounded reality: If pornographic intercourse was truly adultery, and something God takes very seriously; if "real" adultery was something He would not ignore and that Caryn Beth would never be expected to allow to continue in a healthy marriage, then I must, without any compromise, see any and all willful entertainment of pornography as real and as serious as if it were literal adultery. If involvement in actual adultery was unthinkable to me and remained entirely absent from my life, pornographic adultery could also and must also become unthinkable and entirely absent from my life.

Furthermore, Caryn Beth had been entirely blindsided by the revelation of my lengthy involvement with pornography, and of the extensive history of the misuse of my sexuality. For years I had looked her in the face and told her my eyes were for her only. The shocking truth of my duplicity now hit her like a hammer, shattering her trusting, loving, faithful heart into a million pieces. She was understandably horrified and traumatized by my confessions.

It was weeks before she could sit with me and work toward resolution. But before we could even think about a possible future together, she laid down a new bottom line: "No more porn, ever, or its over between us."

I agreed with her on a new consequence to be put in place as her safeguard: in the same way that Jesus in the scriptures gave a woman whose husband engaged in sexual immorality the right and freedom to leave the marriage, we decided together that further deliberate involvement on my part with pornographic intercourse would be grounds for Caryn Beth to separate from me.

That's a major paradigm-shifting consideration to take away from Matthew 5:27-30. It's straight up, bitter medicine, hard truth. But Jesus indicated that such truth holds the keys to our shackles.

Please understand me: in sharing this section of the story of my transformation, I am not trying to empower a spouse to leave a husband who happens to have tripped up on occasion and seen something he should not have seen. I certainly do not promote divorce and am not promoting divorce, especially over the accidental exposure to pornographic imagery that is becoming almost unavoidable in today's world. Let me make it clear that there is in my understanding a big distinction between one who has been exposed to porn, and one who is deliberately pursuing and engaging in pornographic intimacy. At that time, I was definitely in the latter category, and was asleep to the danger I was in. When Caryn Beth wisely, lovingly drew an uncompromising line in the sand for me—"If you want me, then no more porn!"—it proved to be a powerful and effective wake up call.

Dear reader, my heart is to bring a decisive end to the deception that the willful, ongoing cycle of pursuing interaction with porn should be overlooked, either by yourself or by a merciful spouse. Just what am I saying here? I would hope that you would agree that a believing spouse must not ignore or enable her partner to develop an addiction to alcohol or illicit drug use, or to participate in seances and witchcraft, right? In the same way, if a believing partner is showing ongoing commitment to maintaining a pursuit of pornographic intimacy—that is, maintaining a commitment to an addiction to porn— I am suggesting that bringing drastic efforts into the relationship to awaken the erring partner to the danger of his ways is the loving, godly, severely merciful thing to do. (For excellent advise along these lines, please see Dr. James Dobson's book, <u>Love Must Be Tough</u>)

Guilty hands

That new bottom line ***(pornographic intimacy = real adultery)*** wasn't the only thing God highlighted to me from Matthew's text. Let's look at those red letters again.

"You have heard that it was said to those of old, 'You shall not commit adultery.' But I say to you that whoever looks

at a woman to lust for her has already committed adultery with her in his heart. If your right eye causes you to sin, pluck it out and cast it from you; for it is more profitable for you that one of your members perish, than for your whole body to be cast into hell. And if your right hand causes you to sin, cut it off and cast it from you; for it is more profitable for you that one of your members perish, than for your whole body to be cast into hell." (Matt. 5:27-30)

Right after redefining lust and the objectification of women for us, Jesus immediately makes some amazing statements about the misuse of both eyes *and* hands: "Along the lines of active lust contributing to your being guilty of actual adultery, if your right eye is a part of the lust/adultery mix, then gouge it out rather than have it cause you to go to hell." (Of course, that's my own paraphrase.) Wow! Those were radically stern words. It almost seems to be an overly aggressive reaction, if active lust after all is "just a bad habit" as I'd been told. But it's not. Jesus is saying here that unbridled lust is such a big deal to God that it is directly connected with one going to hell! That's intense!

But it's not the eyes only that are involved. "If your right hand causes you to sin, cut it off and throw it away." Wait a minute: the use of your right eye, and the use of your right hand—in the context of talking about the eternally fatal consequences of lust, what do you think Jesus is referring too? I suggest that Jesus is talking very directly and graphically with men about the danger of lustful gaze mixed with the sensational element of masturbation. He's making sure men connect the dots in this deadly equation: Lust + eyes+ masturbation add up to hell being on one's destination list. (See chapter 9 for more on masturbation)

Let me restate that in order to make sure you catch what I am saying, for this truth is a key motivational passage in the battle against dark intimacy. I have not checked with any scholars on this, but I know the Holy Spirit used this passage to shock me awake to the reality that in Mathew 5 Jesus is clearly warning men that *lust in action, coupled with the act of masturbation*—in other words, deliberate, pornographic intercourse—*is so serious a matter that it literally would be better for you to maim yourself if you cannot otherwise decisively end this sin's dominion over you*. Of course such maiming is not the point encouraged by this passage; but the implication is real and clear to me and must not be downplayed: *unrestrained pornographic intercourse will land you in hell. Jesus is deadly serious about this, and you and I must be very aggressive about this cancer: if you are still struggling with this issue, you must put a decisive end to this sin's dominion in your life.*

If this chapter touches on sexual struggle in your own life and the need for some alterations to be made to your perspective, please stop right now (or schedule some devoted time later) to really sit with the Holy Spirit to review and contemplate your own actions in light of this revelation.

With His help, please embrace Jesus' clear redefining of what pornographic intimacy is—He sees it as actual adultery, and He makes sure we know that adulterers will be judged. If you have been deliberately, habitually engaging with porn, please see that, before God, you are guilty of the sin of adultery and are in need of acknowledging that and repenting from it, or else, according to scripture, you will be judged.

And then after contemplating that step, with God's help, embrace as well Jesus' clear warning of the eternal impact that the unrestrained wandering of your eyes are having on you. According to the Rescuer, your own deliberate, lustful gazing at porn places you in danger of ending up in hell. Again, with His help, acknowledge this and repent from this tremendous deception.

And finally, with the Holy Spirit's help, heed Jesus' clear warning of the eternal impact that the practice of masturbation can have on us. According to the Redeemer, your deliberate, ongoing commitment to stimulate your own solitary sexual climax places you in danger of ending up in hell. His words, not mine! Again, if this is an issue in your life, with His help, acknowledge and repent from it.

Dear reader, I have wept several times in the writing of this manuscript, in part because of the sadness of my own errors and the horror of revisiting the darkness and uncleanliness my life used to be haunted by. But yesterday as I wrote I found I was weeping, not for me, but for you; I really want to see you free, to know that you as well are enjoying the perfect love of God and the unending pleasures that are in His right hand, and the unimaginable things He has prepared for those who love Him. I wept yesterday with the responsibility of my part in your freedom and deliverance, because I am in great travail over the work of birthing a similar rescue in your life from the hell that dominated me for so long. I weep because the chances are real that my best attempts might not be enough to convince you to follow my map to freedom. My grief is that my hours and weeks in effort to communicate to you on these pages here might not have made a statement clear enough to lead you away from the cliff you are running toward. But my hope does not rest in me and my efforts: my hope is in the very real, ongoing, inexhaustible efforts of the One who leaves the 99 to find the single stray. I am giving you here just the roughest scaffolding of my story in hopes that the Holy Spirit can and will use it to build for you an escape from your prison too. Please make the most of it! Please plead with Him to add to my efforts the faithful mercy of His anointed vision, His powerful voice, His transcendent capacity to break through any deception, right there where you are, and right now. He is Truth. And it's Truth that makes us free.

"For we will surely die and become like water spilled on the ground, which cannot be gathered up again. Yet God does not take away a life; but He devises means, so that His banished ones are not expelled from Him."
(2 Samuel 14:14)

Chapter 7 Insidious Design

Ok, enough stories: lets go to *War!*

It was divine revelation that saved me from porn.

I wish you could just take my word for it, and then straight away I could just impart the revelation to you, and you could instantly just apply the lessons I've learned to your situation. Like in the movie, the Matrix, the moment when Neo downloads a fighting program directly into his brain and then looks up and states, "I know Kung Fu!"; I wish impartation were that simple. But for the most part, that's not how it works. So I'm trying to do the work necessary for you to fully understand what I'm saying; you need the formula—the proof— to unlock the equation. I'm really hoping something I've learned will help you.

As a writer and counselor and a man hungry to see my brothers really taste the lasting supernatural liberty I have, by God's grace, walked in, I feel a bit at this point like an unschooled math student during his first semester in geometry, as if I've *found* the answers for the problems given as homework, but don't yet know how I *got* the answers. Please stick with me as I try to sift through my recollection of the spiritual transformation that was taking place, to find sufficient natural words for the supernatural equation that added up to my deliverance.

Here's the bottom line— together, you and I have to succeed in answering the question: Why does porn succeed? And not only *succeed*, but *progress*; why is it such a progressive cancer on our society today? (". . . in our society today"—we'll have to talk about that a little later in the book)

And to make sure this is not just an academic/intellectual exercise, keep reminding yourself as you read that I am trying to get us to ask the question:

why is pornography continuing to succeed
within ***your own life***?

I am tired of the time and attention porn has already stolen from us all: if this is your struggle, then I really want this to be the last book you have to read about pornography and sexual addiction before you finally turn a corner and see its destructive presence totally uprooted from your life and see lasting freedom from its power established in a long-term, sustainable fashion. As already reflected on earlier in this book, God is not just interested in our NOT being overcome with evil; He leads us confidently past that step, into the place of our overcoming evil with good. (I strongly recommend memorizing Romans 12:21.) That's absolutely what the work of Christ makes available to you. So let's get there already! That freedom is what you really need. And it's what I believe you really want. I'm sure it's what *He* really wants—the joy of you walking in your blood-bought freedom from the power of darkness is part of the reward Jesus gets for His suffering. It's what He deserves. And (if you're married) it's what your wife and children deserve.

So let's get back to work on this question: *how is it that pornography is succeeding in getting you to repeatedly do something that you really don't want to do?*

Porn and the supernatural dimension

To answer that specific question, I propose that porn succeeds not by accident, but by design. Porn succeeds because it has an agenda—a hidden agenda. At its core, its engines are driven by a sinister program—like a computer virus—loosed into our operating systems in order to prevent the possibility of the good things God has already said He would do for us and with/through us ever coming to pass. I believe part of porn's aim is actually the interception of prophecy, the possibility of prevention of the Kingdom of heaven advancing on earth. Porn is an effort to frustrate or even eliminate the dreams of God.

Think about that for a moment. (See chapter 13 for a more in-depth explanation of what I mean.)

With sinister ideas behind its airbrushed mask, I propose that porn continues to succeed largely because it operates undetected, even as it is infecting our soul's hard drive. So again, it is one of my chief aims to end the undetected aspect of the presence of darkness behind the offer of pornographic intimacy.

Now let's get something straight here: if you're going to keep up with where I'm going and find yourself out in the wide open spaces of the abundant life that Jesus already secured for you to inherit, you as the reader are going to have to decide to walk with me *by faith*. In the last paragraphs I've made mention of a supernatural dimension of the pornographic agenda. I propose that your freedom is totally linked to your believing that such a reality—a conscious, supernatural, sentient, rational darkness that is right now working on your demise—exists. If for whatever reason you cannot come to grips with there being a supernatural dimension to this issue, then I am afraid I can help you no further. There are no two ways around it: if you can't brook what I am saying about the real darkness that props up pornography, then have a nice time trying to engage the help of legalism, pulling yourself up by your own best natural efforts, while in reality continuing to fondle your sickness and ending up in hell. You need read no further.

I make such strong statements because the Bible is my reality anchor, and the Bible is very clear about what I am saying about the supernatural dimensions of sin. In case deception has already moved you past an awareness of that, lets look at some key texts.

Here are some words of life that you and I need to really digest:

" . . . what the law could not do in that it was weak through the flesh, God did by sending His own Son in the likeness of sinful flesh, on account of sin: He condemned sin in the flesh, that the righteous requirement of the law might be fulfilled in us who do not walk according to the flesh but according to the Spirit. For those who live according to the flesh set their minds on the things of the flesh, but those who live according to the Spirit, (set their minds on) the things of the Spirit. For to be carnally minded (that is, mentally focused only on the material/temporal reality) is death (will kill you), but to be spiritually minded (mindful and focused on spiritual reality) is life and peace. Because the carnal mind is enmity against God; for it is not subject to the law of God, nor indeed can be. So

then, those who are in the flesh cannot please God." (Romans 8: 3-8, my paraphrase in parenthesis.)

In short, the law cannot justify us, nor can it sanctify us—it can't save us and it can't help us overcome our propensity for being dominated by the sin inside of us. Only life *in the Spirit* —that is, supernatural life—can offer hope for breaking the power of sin in us.

1 Peter 5:8-9 picks up the conversation:

"Be sober, be vigilant; because ***your adversary the devil walks about like a roaring lion, seeking whom he may devour****. Resist him, steadfast in the faith, knowing that the same sufferings are experienced by your brotherhood in the world."* Wow—good stuff right there. Can you decide here and now to fully believe it? Can you believe with me that its time to stop kidding yourself—that when you are engaged in pornographic intercourse, you are being devoured by darkness' roaring lion? Wake Up!! "Be sober", says the verse: in the Greek, the words mean "be on watch." "Be vigilant:" in the Greek, literally, "stay awake!" If you, as a christian, are playing with porn it is because you are in a stupor about the danger of being personally stalked and attacked by the devil.

I love that Paul goes on in the text to remind the reader that whatever struggle they are facing is the same struggle their brothers throughout the world are facing. That in itself can give you help and hope: you are not alone!

2 Corinthians 2:10-12 is another important text for this discussion. In a passage where Paul is giving counsel about the role forgiveness plays in relationship, he makes the following statement: *"For whom you forgive anything, I also forgive. For if indeed I have forgiven anything, I have forgiven that one for your sakes in the presence of Christ, lest Satan should take advantage of us; for we are not ignorant of his devices."* I include this text here only because it is clear Paul is indicating that A) satan has devices—strategies devised against our well being; and that B) we can be ignorant of them; C) if we are ignorant of them, satan will use our ignorance to take advantage of us. ***Pornography is obviously a device of satan; identify it as such, and stop being ignorant of it's strategic satanic reality***.

Now again, some of you may be saying, "That's so super elementary—I can't believe you are taking time to point that out." Dear Reader, I do so only because I have counseled far too many believers, even pastors, who are engaged with pornography in some sort of apparent ignorance that they are directly engaging with a satanic device and entity. That's something entirely different than eating too many donuts on a Saturday morning.

We must not forget his official title, this roaring lion: Ephesians 2:2 calls him *"the prince of the power of the air."* In some real way, he has rights to the air waves; and in some very real way, I suggest to you that he is using that right to infect society with supernatural darkness like never before.

Supernatural battle: participation mandatory!

If we will be victorious in our fight for maturity and holiness, we must courageously, aggressively align our faith and understanding that, according to scripture, we are called to fight against satan's efforts, and in fact are already fully equipped for supernatural warfare:

2 Cor. 10:3-6 *". . . though we walk in the flesh (that is, though we are experiencing life as humans, clothed in the material/temporal, or in the natural), we do not war according to the flesh (that is, we do not fight in a strictly natural human manner). For the weapons of our warfare are not carnal (not material) but mighty in God for pulling down strongholds, casting down arguments and every high thing that exalts itself against the knowledge of God, bringing every thought into captivity to the obedience of*

Christ, and being ready to punish all disobedience when your obedience is fulfilled." (parenthesis, my paraphrase)

My brothers, hear, in these verses, our call to battle! Hear, in these verses, our call to Holy War! If you are alive—that is, if you are still walking on earth in a body—there is no option of your not being at war! That in itself is profound. It indicates to me that if you are not fighting, you are already a casualty. *Fighting—and fighting a supernatural enemy—is a very real part of your existence and must become a constant aspect of your mental makeup!*

Paul takes us a step further than just inviting us to an awareness of the war: he indicates clearly here that each of us, in Christ, are battle-ready, equipped with MIGHTY weapons, weapons with specific purposes. His explanation of the purposes for our weaponry is for us our transcendent job description and an amazing vision statement—with these weapons we are to be involved in: A) pulling down spiritual strongholds; B) throwing down arguments; C) ripping down every high thing that exalts itself against the knowledge of God; D) bringing every thought into captivity to the obedience of Christ; and E) being ready to punish all disobedience when our obedience is fulfilled.

Elsewhere (2 Cor. 6:7) Paul mentions the use of the armaments, weapons of righteousness in the right and the left hands that he and his fellow ministers make use of in this supernatural work of overcoming evil with good.

He writes in the same vein in Ephesians 6:12, where it is clearly understood from his words that we ARE in battle; that is not the question. The question is who is our enemy?

The biblical answer is very clear: our enemy is NOT other people. *"We do not wrestle against flesh and blood."* But the clear implication is: *we do wrestle!* The opposite of not wrestling against flesh and blood is not to step into some passive state where "Jesus already did it all." That's a lie. A very real result of the work of Jesus on the cross is that He bought back your will, so that you can now pick it up and enforce, by your choice, the victory that Jesus already won. You and I must embrace daily this reality: wrestling for life is a part of the game outside of Eden's gates. We DO wrestle. We MUST!

Lion hunting

But what do we wrestle against? In answer, the Holy Spirit, writing in Ephesians 6:12, lists a chain of command of supernatural entities that are our enemies: *"(we wrestle) against principalities, against powers, against the rulers of the darkness of this age, against spiritual hosts of wickedness in the heavenly places."* When is the last time that you thought of yourself as someone who wrestles against spiritual hosts of wickedness in heavenly places? But that is what we are clearly called to in our choices!

You must stop agreeing with the mental infection seeded into the airwaves that the devil is in no way a part of your struggle. You must stop thinking that he doesn't exist, or that if he does, he might only be involved in someone else's life—as if maybe he's involved in the work of the coven that meets in the back streets of New Orleans or something, but not in your own life. If you're going to come clean, you are going to do so by recognizing that if you are not actively winning a battle against spiritual darkness, it's because you are already a casualty.

I have to be honest and tell you: its not only the devil who does not want you to live in an awareness of his existence; sometimes, even within the church there is a spirit of religion that is also very much involved in helping you deny the reality of the supernatural dimension of sin.

I mentioned briefly early in the book that I was born again when I was 16. As soon as the revelation of the beautiful love of God captured my heart, I gave my life to Him right there and then, and decided that all I wanted to do was go to bible school where I could study scripture in the original languages and thereby get as close to knowing God as possible. So two years later, I graduated from high school and off I went to a conservative Bible college, where I enrolled as a pre-seminary Bible major with a minor in psychology. It was there that in a class on Angelology and Demonology, I was formally taught by a brilliant scholar in Hebrew, Greek and Aramaic, that demons are no longer present in the world. Hmmm. What great news! I ate it up.

I'm not going to take on those findings here from an academic standpoint—that is, I'm not going to try and look at that professor's research and find out if his conclusions were *correct*. I am, instead, going to give you real world experience that must ask whether or not that professor's conclusions were *true*. I propose that they were not. My 5 year old daughter convinced me of as much.

Demon in my home

We were living in Kenya for less than a year when our daughter turned 5. Being up above the clouds for hours during the long flight from New York to Nairobi, it was her first time to really contemplate heaven. Later, she had asked her mom all about where God lived; that tender conversation led into a simple explanation of the gospel, and Rachel had been born again. At the time, we were, as I've indicated, pretty conservative believers, and had very little, if any, real exposure to the supernatural, or to deliverance or exorcism. It was therefore a great surprise to us one evening when Rachel began screaming in her bedroom: "Get out, in Jesus' Name! Get out, in Jesus Name!" Her mother and I rushed in to calm her from what we thought must be a bad dream. But Rachel was wide awake and adamant: "I was not dreaming mom—I was still awake! I saw something at the end of my bed. It looked like a pig and it had red eyes, and it just stared at me, and I knew it was bad! And when I shouted, 'Get out in Jesus name', it left!"

Rachel was never one to make things up, never one to exaggerate, never one to lie. Gentle questioning led us both to the conclusion that Rachel had indeed seen "something"; the only explanation we could come up with was that the "something" had been supernatural. That she had been able to identify it as such was a puzzle to me; that she had needed to and had known specifically how to effectively drive it out of her room left me shaken. I cannot help but wonder what would have happened in that interaction if she had not had the Holy Spirit's guidance, now so readily available to her young heart and mind since she had just been born again and He had taken up residence in her precious little heart.

This (and several other equally eye-opening and otherwise unexplainable supernatural encounters that we experienced first hand in Africa) eventually convinced me that my prof in college did not have the full picture. I feel, in fact, that his teaching that demons are no longer active in the earth actually feeds into the very hand the devil wants to play: that is, that he wants us to think that he does not really exist (or at least is no where near our existence) and therefore we don't need to be so concerned about his influence. Paul writes to the young pastor, Timothy, that *" . . . the Spirit expressly says that in latter times some will depart from the faith, giving heed to deceiving spirits and doctrines of demons."* (1 Timothy 4:1)

Impotence in the last days

A world devoid of the belief in present supernatural powers of darkness is only the flip side of a christian life similarly disempowered. The two are inseparable. I believe it is an end-time doctrine from hell that teaches that supernatural darkness and light are theoretical, historical considerations — like the study of dinosaurs or Neanderthal man—that although interesting, have little impact on our present reality. This is a hell-spawned lie that I embraced and one I feel made room for darkness to secretly invade my life for far too long. *This lie must be rooted out of your mind if you are to overcome the dominion of pornography in your life.*

The Bible warns us about an impotent end-times people, one that has a form of godliness but that at the same time, denies its power (2 Timothy 3:5). As I mentioned earlier in this book, in my search for help from several conservative, secessionist pastors, I could not find any who understood or even acknowledged the supernatural dimension behind my actions. And so they had no effective help to offer me. Someone finally offered me the book, The Bondage Breaker, by Neil Anderson. This was a huge game-changer for me and turned out to be the source of my deliverance. After such a long and fruitless search for help in my battle, I could sense even in just the first few pages of Neil's work, the liberating power of the Truth it contained. As I started to read it, for the first time I began to see that maybe I could be set free. Excitedly, I shared my hope with the conservative man who was my pastor at the time. He was one of the several to whom I'd confessed my struggles and was asking for help. "I think Neil Andersons' work is a bunch of bunk!" He replied. It was then that he turned to me, looked me squarely in the eyes and said with very palpable disdain: "Our prisons are lined with double-minded christians like you. You're never going to change. I'm keeping my eye on you!" (And of course he never did—I literally never heard from him again.)

Although the words I heard were so painful, I so appreciate that God allowed that pastor to really overplay his cards that day; in my opinion, this man was blind, like the Pharisees of Jesus day. In encountering the Pharisees' role in the lives of those of their disciples who were honestly trying to find God, Jesus said of such shepherds:

"Leave them; they are blind leaders of the blind. And if the blind leads the blind, both will fall into a ditch."
(Matt. 15:14 NIV)

That day in the face of such a statement of loveless judgement and condemnation from my pastor, I was able to answer in grace and say this: "From what I've read so far in this book (that you say is bunk), I think Jesus just might know what to do to set me free. So I am going to trust in Him and see where that takes me." Then I turned and walked away. I soon left that church. To find my healing, I had to leave the blind guides I was familiar with. From that moment on, God led me onward in the (still ongoing) discovery of the entire supernatural dimension of life. (FYI: Neil Anderson's, The Bondage Breaker, is the one book I continue to use with so many who are searching for help with any number of addictive issues. I cannot overstate its value in making room for unplugging deception. I strongly recommend you get a copy and go through it, and then keep it as a reference in your own library for others in need of help. In addition to the revelatory encounters I was having with the Holy Spirit, Neil's book was all I had as I sought for deliverance; but it was enough to see me through to final freedom from darkness.)

Do you really believe?

Perhaps you are at the place of needing similar help. You must choose as well to stop living in ignorance of the supernatural dimension of life, and the supernatural dimension of sin. You must choose to believe in the present reality of darkness, infecting the airwaves, attempting to cloud your conscience, and blind your vision. You too MUST BELIEVE. And in fact, I am not talking about only believing in the devil; if you want to see real change come to you in your fight to control your own body, you must come to fully believe *in God*.

I'll never forget the day that the Spirit of God challenged me with this statement: *"You don't really believe in me."*

"What?!!! Of course I do!" was my strong, immediate reply.

"No, you don't!"

What do you do when God steps close to your ears and tells you that you don't believe in Him? And how important is the answer to that question?

Chapter 8 Believing is Seeing

Early 1999

"You don't really believe," God said to me one day. *"Not really. You're not really a christian, like you think you are. And you need to understand that."*

1999 was the year transformational awakening really began to take place in me. Bit by bit, the Holy Spirit had been walking me into what real repentance needed to look like, as He prepared me for a whole new life of faithfulness and a commitment to the purity and consecration that had always been His dream for my existence. But before I was ready to become *really* born again (again!) He needed to talk me through my unbelief.

When He said to me point blank that from His perspective, I was not a believer, I was confused. *"What do you mean?"* I asked. His answer was profound: *"When you choose to walk into a gas station to buy gas and encounter unexpectedly that they sell porn, and you end up purchasing a Playboy magazine, you are making that choice based on the faulty thinking that no one will see what you're doing. Although I can see that the action of making such a purchase makes you nervous, you also act in confidence as if I am not aware of what you are doing. At the same time, I know you are at least familiar with words I have stated that make it clear that I see all, and that there will come a day when you will have to give an account for everything that you do in private. When you act as if I do not exist, in some very real sense, from my perspective, I am telling you that you do not believe in me."*

He was right. I could see that at such times, although I knew Him to be who He is, I was trading that transcendent reality—truth— for my choice to meet my selfish desire for immediate comfort (or whatever falsehood of the day I was fondling). I was in fact deliberately *ignoring reality*. When I did this, I was un-believing, literally *undoing belief*. And in the cycle I was in, of choosing un-belief over and over and over, I was putting myself into a dangerous position where, at some core level, God was defining me as a non-believer.

I was quiet for a long time, mulling this over. Again, like a truly caring Father, God was trying to make an important point, and the tip of His quick and powerful, two-edged sword was cutting deep through the levels of deception I had become so comfortable with.

He continued: *"If you are going to truly walk away from the sins of your youth, you are going to do so by stepping into the reality of living with a constant awareness of my presence."*

Practicing the presence of my family

I distinctly remember that at this moment in the dialogue, I balked. *"I don't know how to do that . . . I can't see you, I can't feel you—how can I live with a constant awareness of your presence?"* (I remembered a phrase from a book I had read by Brother Lawrence, about 'Practicing the Presence of God.' In spite of my having read the book, I had obviously not been very good at the practice.)

His answer was inspiring and simple: *"Imagine that in order to pick up a dozen eggs, you are going to walk into a 7/11, where you know they sell pornography. If you had your wife, and your young son and daughter with you, holding your hands, would you walk over together and also purchase a Playboy?"*

"No way!" I replied: *"of course not!".*

"Of course not. Good. What makes the difference?"

"The presence of my family. I would be far too ashamed to make such a purchase with their full knowledge of what I was doing."

Moment of truth; He continued: *"Some day—some real actual day— they will see all that you are doing, and all that you have ever done. None of it will be whitewashed. All will be plainly visible. And in some timeless way, you need to make that awareness a part of your decision making processes, moment by moment."*

Then came a stellar idea from His brilliant mind and tender heart: *"If it is difficult at this point for you to practice My presence and an awareness of eternity, why don't you start to practice the constant presence of your family—pretend that no matter where you go, you go together—all of you, all the time, together. Like a game of pretend. Can you do that?"*

I said I would try. And try I did. And my world began to change. Immediately.

I am sorry if I am not fully capable of explaining what transpired as I set out on this new experiment, but what took place was some sort of supernatural alteration of my mental programming: although still on earth, locked in the maze of commonplace ins and outs of life, as I started to imagine that my family was now always with me, I began to also be aware of eternity—of my spiritual existence beyond life on earth, in time, and space— in a way I had never before been aware. The practice of the presence of my own family really worked: when I, all alone, encountered a tempting well-orchestrated invitation for me to side-step reality and slide back into bad choices, I said to myself that no, I couldn't do that, because my family was (invisibly) with me and would see me doing it, and that was just an unthinkable thought. I let myself be moved by the shame that would hit me if I had revealed to my family that I was still choosing to delve into the depths of depravity. I told myself that my family really *was* with me in my truck as I drove alone to work and back, was with me on my solitary lunch breaks, was with me when I stopped for gas or groceries, alone, when I got off work at 11:30 pm.

And actually, it was not very long before my heart and mind made the seamless jump from my easily, constantly practicing the presence of my family, to my constantly practicing the transcendent presence of God. From that point on, I *was never alone*. I realize now that I AM NEVER ALONE! And as a result, *I never purchased pornography again!*

This was not entirely the end of my war, but it was definitely the end of the dominion of immediacy over my mindset: soon the practice of the presence of God became an easy addition to my expanding and freshly cleansed operating system, where eternity was my new awareness normal, and holiness was becoming a friend and beloved companion, instead of a dreaded judge and an impossibility. (More on that topic in chapter 14)

Altered state of mind

Because this long-awaited transformation in me was suddenly so easily administered, I want to make room for the same to take place in you. To do so I want to share the powerful truth of scripture. The writer of Hebrews makes this point: "*. . . the word of God is living and powerful, and sharper than any two-edged sword, piercing even to the division of soul and spirit, and of joints and marrow, and is a discerner of the thoughts and intents of the heart. And there is no creature hidden from His sight, but all things are naked and open to the eyes of Him to whom we must give account.*" (Hebrews 4:12-13)

You will remember my aim is not so much to teach you, to inform your mind. My aim is to reach with Truth's liberating touch those of you who are continuing to sin because you have willfully invited deception into your minds. Scripture says sin weighs heavily on us, and easily tangles us in its chains. If you are weighed down with sin's deception, I want to bring the truth into such inner chambers of your existence and break off any chains that might have entangled you.

The Word of God ***is living***. Another translation says the Word of God is ***ALIVE!*** The Word of God is also ***POWERFUL!*** It is shaped and capable of cutting through the crap—the refuse of all the devil's work of blinding our eyes and infecting our operating systems. Let's take a moment to look at the living, power-filled truths in the scriptures that undergird the things God was, like a tender dad, revealing to me:

Numbers 32:23b " *. . . take note, (when) you have sinned against the Lord; and be sure your sin will find you out."* You and I must choose to truly believe that this is true.

Ecc. 12:13-14: *"Let us hear the conclusion of the whole matter: Fear God and keep His commandments, for this is man's all. For God will bring every work into judgment, including every secret thing, whether good or evil."* Again, we must choose to *believe* that this is absolutely true!

Luke 8:17 *"For nothing is secret that will not be revealed, nor anything hidden that will not be known and come to light."* Guess what? (Again:) You and I must choose to believe that this is really, fully true!

Luke 12: 2-3: *"For there is nothing covered that will not be revealed, nor hidden that will not be known.Therefore whatever you have spoken in the dark will be heard in the light, and what you have spoken in the ear in inner rooms will be proclaimed on the housetops."*

Romans 2:5-11: *"But in accordance with your hardness and your impenitent heart you are treasuring up for yourself wrath in the day of wrath and revelation of the righteous judgment of God, who 'will render to each one according to his deeds': eternal life to those who by patient continuance in doing good seek for glory, honor, and immortality; but to those who are self-seeking and do not obey the truth, but obey unrighteousness—indignation and wrath, tribulation and anguish, on every soul of man who does evil, of the Jew first and also of the Greek; but glory, honor, and peace to everyone who works what is good, to the Jew first and also to the Greek. For there is no partiality with God."*

1 Peter 4:3-5: *"For we have spent enough of our past lifetime in doing the will of the Gentiles—when we walked in lewdness, lusts, drunkenness, revelries, drinking parties, and abominable idolatries. In regard to these . . . (all) will give an account to Him who is ready to judge the living and the dead."*

Soon, all will see and know all

All of this is true and if we are going to see transformation come to our darkest areas, we must choose to believe and permit these truths to reform our reality. I take the time to bring all these verses to our attention because they were the backdrop for the kindness of God coming to me and warning me about my own unbelief. These verses are unshakably true, and are now my unalterable reality: they are a part of the very scaffolding of my existence. God sees, and knows, and soon all will see all, and all will know. The idea that we might escape this reality is an indication of our having broken with reality. There is no secret; there's nothing I've ever done wrong that somehow slipped through the cracks, unnoticed. Some day you will see all the wrong I have done, and I will see all the wrong you have done. For me that translated into the fact that some day my innocent children and precious wife would know my greatest errors. Contemplation of this shocking aspect of my future moved me to lasting change.

Dear Reader, please hear behind all of this only the tremendous kindness of the Father. He was concerned enough about the practices that were fueled by my unbelief that He broke through the space and time continuum and bluntly told me I was *NOT* a believer! This was a shocking consideration to me. But of course, it turns out that God knew what He was saying; I was living in unbelief, regardless of my confession of faith. He was casting a new vision for me; He was inviting me to BELIEVE!

Mulling all of this over for days, I finally came to see for the first time in my life that God is not so focused as I had supposed on whether or not I had once prayed a particular prayer, or had called myself a christian, or that I thought of myself as someone who had been "born again." He was, however, fundamentally concerned with and deadly serious about someone coming to believe in the supernatural aspects of their own existence, of the supernatural existence of evil, and especially of the supernatural existence of God Himself. He was interested in belief. And He was explaining to me that *unbelief* was at the source of my continuing to do things that by now, I was no longer interested in doing but could not figure out how to stop doing them. He was explaining that **in that battle, *belief was going to be key*.**

As I have indicated off and on through this story so far, in light of my pornographic preoccupation, the possibility of my going to hell had become a part of my concerned thoughts; but now I was beginning to understand that I would not go to hell because I was into porn—*IF* I went to hell, it would be because I chose porn and sex and comfort and pain avoidance as my domain, my dominant reality, instead of believing in the very present reality of a loving God who was interested in constant, interactive, personal relationship with me. *Belief* was what God was whispering to me as being of primary importance, belief that was so deeply entwined with my very heart and will that because of it, I would walk out all my days with a proper respect for Him—what the scriptures call *the fear of God*— and unswerving appreciation of life as He suggested it be lived, and consequent obedience to His directions. This is the life of faith God was inviting me into.

I cannot tell you how much my heart is wed to the writing of this book, laying the groundwork for the overwhelmingly beautiful work that Jesus loves to do, in bringing hope into shadows, planting fields of flowers in former wastelands. Working on this chapter yesterday, I wrote until late into the night, overextending my bedtime by at least an hour. The next morning, although I hungered again to jump back into this manuscript, I felt instead that the writing should wait until I was done with my regular time of scripture reading and mediation. Believing it to be better to start the day with an appropriate foundation of "fresh bread" than to just run on my own fumes with the project I was passionate about, I opened my iPhone and scrolled to my reading schedule, and then started reading the first of three pre-assigned chapters from the Bible. That first assignment was from John 6. Reading along in the chapter that starts with Jesus feeding of the 5000, I felt immediately transported, and enjoyed a welcome reprieve from the focus of the topics in my writing.

However, as the chapter scrolled on, I suddenly found myself reading material that I know Heaven was orchestrating to fit right back into this chapter of Holy. War. and the very topic of the importance of real belief. (I SOOO LOVE it when the very present Helper leans over my shoulders and does that!!)

The ONE important thing: you gotta believe!

In John 6, the text records that crowds of people who were honestly interested in knowing how to please God, approached Jesus with the very question we, with other words, have been trying to ask here in this book: 'What do we have to do in order to be right with God?' Here's what the dialogue sounded like (with my simple paraphrase of the conversation in parenthesis):

John 6:28-29: *"What shall we do, that we may work the works of God?" Jesus answered and said to them, "This is the work of God, that you believe in Him whom He sent."* (This is God's top priority, the ONE issue that you have to clearly understand and embrace: *you have to believe in Him*.)

The religious crowd, used to a list of "do"s and "don't"s in their efforts to gain divine favor, is skeptical of that "simple" answer. Sifting through their faith levels, Jesus is very straightforward with the doubters about why He has an issue with them:

6:36: *"I said to you that you have seen Me and yet do not believe."* (In spite of your privileged access to me, you still don't take me at my word: Belief in Me is *THE* issue. You can't skip around that and still keep going forward on any level in your attempt to reach God.)

6:40: *" . . . this is the will* (the choice, the inclination, the desire, the pleasure) *of Him who sent Me* (that is, this is what the Father really wants): *that everyone who sees the Son and believes in Him may have everlasting life; and I will raise him up at the last day."* (Here's the bottom line: Your being *fully alive,* on every level—forever— is my father's real, chief desire; and belief in me is the doorway to that level of endless, fullest existence, the existential doorway to real supernatural life, the spiritual life that will not end, even with the seeming finality of death.")

6:47: *"Most assuredly, I say to you, he who believes in Me has everlasting life."*

6:55-57: *"My flesh is food indeed, and My blood is drink indeed. He who eats My flesh and drinks My blood abides in Me, and I in him. As the living Father sent Me, and I live because of the Father, so he who feeds on Me will live because of Me."* (Look: you must make the reality of 'Me' your fundamental understanding of vitality; My existence must move beyond the theological, beyond the academic, and beyond the intellectual: I must become the very body in which you are alive, the pulsing revenant corpse you exist in and from. Through faith, My life must become your life, must transcend your life—our lives must flow together inseparably.)

6:63b, 64 *"The words that I speak to you are spirit, and they are life. But there are some of you who do not believe." For Jesus knew from the beginning who they were who did not believe, and who would betray Him."*

Wow. This final verse really hit me this morning: even now, as Jesus looks down on your life and all He knows about your choices, He knows who really are just fooling themselves, those who say they are christians—or pastors, or worship leaders, or whatever—but in reality do not believe, *and who would betray Him.*

You cannot continue to both pretend you believe and also deny Him with your choices, and yet not end up

***betraying Him in the end. Please take this warning very seriously*.

6:66: *"From that time many of His disciples went back and walked with Him no more."*

This issue of choosing to have true belief be the dividing line in your day-to-day private life and actions, is the very point at which many may choose to turn away from faith. It is my prayer that it is the very point at which many of you are deeply convicted, perhaps for the first time truly aware of the depth of God's awareness of the games you have been playing, and of your own need to confess and renounce the dominant unbelief that now you need to expel, embracing real faith in its place, and entering into life in Christ by faith.

Please allow that the Holy Spirit just inserted all of that from John 6, in an attempt to highlight the centrality of BELIEF. Please allow me again to speak with both the tenderest, compassionate, invitational voice, and a very bold, serious warning: *until your belief in God becomes the most transcendent framework of your constant reality, sin will likely remain in dominion over you, and you well may end up alone, and cast out of the presence of the Holy God, who only ever wanted you to be well, to be whole, to be ALIVE, FOREVER*.

God's shocking statement, *"You don't really believe . ."* was an invitation to me to really look my own faith in the mirror. That experience brought me to a place of my choosing to BELIEVE, and it was this real belief and the transcendent awareness of eternity that came with it which brought a lasting end to my long affair with pornography.

A final scripture for this chapter: this morning, after my reading in John 6, my iPhone schedule directed me to begin reading James chapter 1. So after being delightfully surprised that the Spirit of God had woven John 6 into this chapter, I was not surprised when I read the following in James:

James 1:6b-8: *". . . he who doubts is like a wave of the sea driven and tossed by the wind. For let not that man suppose that he will receive anything from the Lord; he is a double-minded man, unstable in all his ways."*

Time for doubt to die

"Doubt" is the practice of calling into question the truth of something. In that sense, in relation to the topic of this chapter, I felt like the Holy Spirit was again showing up at my desk and whispering in my ear again, effectively influencing the writing of this chapter with these verses from James. Basically, in reading them, I hear for you again the echo of what He was saying to me back in '99: *"Let's shatter any illusions right here and now. You can't live in doubt of My reality any longer—that is, you can't safely deny My realty through your choices of lesser reality any longer. Its time for a decisive end to double-mindedness. You have to embrace the truth that you cannot 'have your cake and eat it too' any longer—you cannot call yourself a 'believer' and hold the office of ambassador of the kingdom of God while at the same time living as if I do not really exist and as if My very serious warnings about what you do in secret really don't apply to you and your little privileged life. Double-mindedness will suck the life out of you. It will make you an unbeliever. And unbelievers end up in the lake of fire."*

You can decide today: you can come clean, or you can keep pretending, keep un-believing; in the end, you will be found out. There is no escaping the Truth.

So how about we come clean right here and now?! Today is a great day for Freedom to spread! If you feel ready for it, I've written below a sample prayer for you to pray:

"Holy Spirit, I invite the fullness of the life and power of Your word to be wholly active in me! I call its life into effective action here and now in this war over my own life.

With my own mouth, with my own will, I hereby resist the devil by inviting the living and powerful word of God to come, in all its focused, sharp capacity, to cut through any deception that has kept me locked in temporal thought patterns, and in false concepts of whether or not I could escape Your notice, my God, of my wrong choices. I freely, gladly, humbly acknowledge that I need Your help in order to renew my mind and step into the constant awareness of eternity. I need Your help in order to step into the awareness of Your constant presence. For my deliverance and well being, and with the help and under the blood of my crucified and risen savior, Jesus Christ, I deliberately renounce the priority of the immediate—the temporal—the material—and I renew my mind with the beautiful, inescapable reality of eternity. I hereby renounce the lie that I exist in any sort of isolation, and I hereby embrace the reality that I am surrounded by a great cloud of witnesses. I renounce the lie that I have ever lived or could ever live one millisecond outside of the presence of God and I hereby choose to consciously live in the continued awareness of my ever-present Helper. Holy Spirit, activate all these truths in me on every level, even as I trust and rest completely in You."

Chapter 9 The Smile in the Dark

By this point in my journey to wholeness, I had finally turned a big corner in my private world. Over the course of approximately two years of very well-orchestrated turbulence, God had graciously delivered to me the bread crumb trail that led to the recovery/liberation of my own will. For the first time since I had first been exposed to it in my teens, I was seeing through the lie of porn's marketing, and was therefore, of my own volition, finally saying "no" to the false intimacy pornography offered. This was huge. But I was soon to realize that porn was not the only ingredient in the narcotic that had been my go-to coping mechanism for dealing with discomfort in my life and my fear of facing responsibility. If I was to really enter into wholeness, I needed to identify and diffuse pornography's partner in crime: I needed to face my need to be done with masturbation.

The realization came to me in a very unorthodox manner. I was still working through the renewing of my mind from the years of processing challenges with the mind of the flesh. On one particular day, I was feeling pretty low; I don't recall what difficulty I'd encountered. I only recall that for the first time, instead of reaching for porn *and* masturbation in order to feel better, I knew I had to plot a *new* coarse toward the comfort I was desperate for at the moment. After all I'd learned and the grounds gained in recent weeks, I could not, in good conscience, turn to porn any longer; but I was in a significant enough level of personal need for comfort/pain avoidance/fear that I locked myself into the windowless bathroom of our apartment, shut off the lights, rolled a towel to block out the light beneath the door and slipped off my clothes. In the total darkness, once again under the illusion that I was really alone, I proceeded to pleasure myself.

I knew it (masturbation) was wrong. I hated myself for heading down what I already knew was a dead-end. I despised where I was going, but I was in too much pain to face whatever it was that was haunting me at the time.

However, before I reached the ecstasy that I was gunning for, there, in the inky blackness, I was shocked and totally unhorsed by the sudden awareness that I was not, as I had suspected, alone in the small room. How did I know this? I knew it because suddenly, in the pitch dark, I saw the pure white teeth of the smile of Perfect Love.

I only "saw" these teeth—this beautiful smile— for a fraction of a second. And the teeth of the smile were all I saw. Nothing else. But in that instantaneous revelation I knew what I had seen was real. And I knew whom that smile belonged to: somehow in my spirit man, I knew I had been allowed to see the smile of Jesus.

I was overwhelmed. I had been trying to raise the bar on my character, but here I was at a very low moment, wrapped in the intensely personal, disgusting attire of wrong, literally caught with my pants down, my own primal selfishness naked very exposed to the eyes of Him to whom nothing is hidden; yet, even in my tremendous weakness, God found a way to totally blow away the size of my comparatively insignificant weakness with the transcendence of His calm, steady, deliberate love. Even in my darkest moment, He was still chasing me down, still inviting me to an intimacy and a real embrace that was bigger/purer/more comforting than anything I could attain on my own.

It was not that my sin meant nothing to Him; it's just that He knew I was still seeing my own need as this impenetrably strong tower, the largest, most unshakable thing in my world. Jesus knew better. His smile revealed that His Love was incomparably stronger than my deepest need.

Transcendent affection: doorway to intimacy

It was the seeing of this Smile of His that really ended it all for me, ended my immaturity and partnering with the preeminence of need. This was the moment on this journey that overabundant forgiveness—on the deepest possible level— was truly manifest to me. It was a forgiveness that went far beyond whatever I was doing at that moment—it was offered to wipe away the power and stain of all the wrong I had ever done. My sin had appeared impossibly huge; but His grace was so much greater. Paul said it this way: *". . . where sin abounded, grace abounded much more!"* (Romans 5:20b)

At that moment, still naked there in the dark bathroom, I stepped past my shame, and stopped what I was doing. And I fell in love with God.

I fell. In love. With God.

There really are no better words to describe what took place. At my worst moment, Jesus had supernatural shown up and smiled at me as if I was His pure and spotless child/follower/disciple/lover. There was such total confidence—such certainty of the choice He'd made to love me, all conveyed in His smile; there was no worry about what He was getting in the deal. He knew full well what He was doing in smiling at me so. I did not have to be offered such grace a second time; I took that radiant smile and ran with it. 21 years later now, I run with it still.

In an amazing story in Luke 7, over dinner in the home of a reserved, self-righteous Pharisee, Jesus explains the unashamed emotional outpouring of affection that a former prostitute was right then and there displaying for Him. Such a lavish exhibit of tenderness is simple to explain, Jesus points out, because the one expressing such affection is one who has been forgiven an impossibly large debt; he or she who has been forgiven much, loves much. (Luke 7:47b: *"to whom little is forgiven, the same loves little."*) 2000 years later and 6,500 miles from the sight of that dinner, I, having received in that dark bathroom, perfect absolution, turned my heart completely over in love to God.

Masturbation was an issue that from time to time would appear at my door, testing my newfound resolve, seeing if I might be talked back into bed with self-soothing; but by the grace of God found in His smile in the darkness, from that time on I no longer made love to myself. After years of having been dominated and tormented by the ecstasy and shame of this cycle of romancing shadows, this final chain had been broken.

From time to time, Jesus has a way of showing up and changing people's names: Abram becomes Abraham. Sarai, Sarah. Jacob, Israel. Cephas, Peter. It was soon after this moment in my development that I sensed His invitation for me to step into a change of my own name: up until that point, all of my 37 years I had been called Jeff. But with this final change in my heart, my very name became a doorway to testifying about the supernatural transformation that was taking place: I stepped into the fullness of my name and started telling people my name was Jeffrey: Jeff-who-is-Free.

Freed from a powerful master

Before we move on from this topic, I want to take a few minutes and take a new look at what is going on when someone orchestrates ecstasy with themselves. Not exactly an everyday conversation, but we need to talk enough that any and all dragons are disrobed and dismissed from your life and mine, alright?!

I want to approach this conversation from the perspective of what I felt the Holy Spirit was bringing to my attention, so let me take us to 1 Corinthians 6:12-20. Lets read through the text as three separate chunks, and tear into each chunk along the way:

"All things are lawful for me, but all things are not helpful. All things are lawful for me, but I will not be brought under the power of any. Foods for the stomach and the stomach for foods, but God will destroy both it and them. Now the body is not for sexual immorality but for the Lord, and the Lord for the body. And God both raised up the Lord and will also raise us up by His power." (1 Cor. 6:12-14)

There are perhaps many christians (even gifted pastors and counselors, as I found out) who really dance around the whole issue of self-soothing, some who may even argue that masturbation is not specifically outlawed in scripture. It sure could have been, by the All-Wise, right? But it wasn't. What does that mean? Well, whatever it *COULD* mean to us all, for me this scripture helped straighten out the mind-gaming possibilities, saying to me that: {the following is my paraphrase as pertains to this discussion}

"Even IF masturbation is lawful for me to engage in, and even IF there is the slightest possibility that it is in some way helpful (as a psychological coping mechanism) (an idea which I confidently DO NOT entertain), ***I must not be brought under the power of it.*** *I must not let it corner me into submission to it as my master. (Interesting that at least in English, the term, masturbate, starts with the phonetic equivalent of Master). This must not be my Master. I have been there, to the place of its dominion over me, and felt the oppressive enslavement of it, and I must not allow that to be the case any more."*

Here again, I paraphrase: *"Eventually, both the body and sexuality will be a thing of the past—God will destroy them both.* ***We will transcend them****. For the here and now, we must anchor our understanding and actions to this truth:*

the body is not meant for sexual immorality, but for intimacy with the Lord. And the Lord is meant for intimacy with the body. And the same way that God raised the Lord up, causing Him to transcend common human existence, He will also raise us up by His power. Turning away from the dominion of masturbation and the 'right' to sooth oneself, is turning toward the coming transcendence. Saying no to masturbation is a part of our being raised up by God's power."

Let's read the next section from the original text:

"Do you not know that your bodies are members of Christ? Shall I then take the members of Christ and make them members of a harlot? Certainly not! Or do you not know that he who is joined to a harlot is one body with her? For "the two," He says, "shall become one flesh." But he who is joined to the Lord is one spirit with Him."
(1 Cor. 6:15-17)

Touching the body parts of Jesus

My paraphrase again: *"Aren't you aware that your bodies are the very limbs/body parts of Christ? Shall I then, in such a thoughtless, inconsiderate manner, dismember a part of Christ and graft it together with someone else, someone who is sexually enslaved by darkness? No way!*

But this is what I do, if I take part in masturbation and pornographic intimacy—it is as if I am actually uniting with sexually enslavement; and my doing so is as if forcing Christ to join me in uniting with deep, dark depravity. This can't be: my being one with Christ—truly being united to Him—means I have married, as it were, His Holy Spirit. Imagine the horrific discomfort the Holy Spirit feels if I ignore His Presence inside of me, and force Him to unite with depravity through pornographic/intimate climax!"

The original text goes on:

"Flee sexual immorality. Every sin that a man does is outside the body, but he who commits sexual immorality sins against his own body. Or do you not know that your body is the temple of the Holy Spirit who is in you, whom you have from God, and you are not your own? For you were bought at a price; therefore glorify God in your body and in your spirit, which are God's." (1 Cor. 6:18-20)

My thoughts: *"Dear brothers, run from this issue! This sin is in a category unlike other addictive sins: for in a way, sexual sin forces union between a vessel in which the Holy Spirit is encased and a vessel that is filled with the toxins of hell. The resulting caustic nature of bringing light and darkness into forced contact* ***will harm your own body!***

And by the way: ***never forget that your body****, the very place where the Holy God of the universe has humbly committed Himself to living inside of—for the sake of your having Comfort reside inside of you—* ***DOES NOT BELONG TO YOU! Your life —the purchase price of your freedom from your former slave master—was very expensive and its freedom has been paid for in full! You have been redeemed! Never forget the significance of that truth. So honor your new Owner, in and with your body, and in and with your spirit, both of which belong to God."***

Dismiss masturbation. End its role in offering help. Whatever part it has played in your inner world, God is now calling you higher and empowering your ascension. Decide that from now on, ecstasy is something you will never taste of alone, never something you will drink from without the Holy Spirit fully present.

Lets close this chapter with acknowledging the great hope set before you: I am 56 years old now, and I have been free from pornographic intimacy for 21 years. After having spent years under the addictive dominion of its deception, by the grace and mercy of Christ, and by following the breadcrumbs left by the Bread of Life, I was able to stop submitting to the fascination I had with pornography.

Having encountered Perfect Love in the midst of a dark moment of shame, I was able to dismiss my use of self-soothing/masturbation and step into a higher calling. We will look for the remainder of this book at some of the ways that the Holy Spirit has coached my walking out these liberating choices. But for now please know that freedom is real and is available to you! By the blood (and brilliant smile) of the Lamb, I am an overcomer. And if I can be one, you can be one too!

Chapter 10 Naked and Unashamed

Remember, my brothers, that this book has been written in tremendous hopes of my giving you some means of aggressively helping yourself get out of the cycle of sin that you have been trying to rid yourself of. It is my sole objective that this book would help you, as Hebrews 12 starts out, to *"throw off everything that hinders and the sin that so easily entangles."* My prayer is that my story will somehow inspire you to *"run with perseverance that race that has been marked out for us."* (Both quotes are from Hebrews 12:1-2 NIV)

As we've looked at so far, in the race I had been called to run, I had finally turned a big corner on my captivating sins and was stepping into freedom. I had been tenderly, earnestly, patiently schooled by the Holy Counselor into finally seeing my sin as it really was; I had walked past the draw of porn and the coping mechanism of masturbation, thrown off the label of "coward" and faced my need to embrace courage and stop running from challenges. I'd become a *real Believer* on this journey, and stepped into a constant awareness of eternity and the Eternal One, my Ever Present. Proudly bearing my new name, I was, in truth, finally turning about face from my sin cocktail and was walking steadily in a new direction.

This is what true repentance is. And this is what Jesus often called out: *REPENT—turn entirely around in your way of thinking and head the other way, for the Kingdom of Heaven is now at hand!* (See Matthew 4:17)

That statement is so important I am going to restate it: Repent! Turn your heart around and head in an entirely new direction, because whatever petty earth-bound mindset and sins you are entangled with are keeping you from being engaged with the very kingdom of heaven. This call to repentance is a joyful sound, an exciting invitation, a call to more than you can imagine: this is the cheer that points us to life: *REPENT!!!*

We all know that stopping sin, confessing, and turning from it, are one thing: walking out that repentance over time is another altogether. By the grace of God, empowering my redeemed will, I have now walked out that repentance for the last twenty one years. And I feel the Holy Spirit wants me to share some of the helpful empowering little tweaks to my reality that were necessary in order for me to remain the pure new man that I had finally been set free to be.

In this same pursuit, Paul instructs his readers in the vital necessity of *taking every thought captive to the obedience of Christ.* (See 2 Corinthians 10:5). He writes elsewhere, encouraging the same disciplined efforts by saying this: *"You know that in a race all the runners run, but only one gets the prize. So run to win! All those who compete in the games use self-control so they can win a crown. That crown is an earthly thing that lasts only a short time, but our crown will never be destroyed. So I do not run without a goal. I fight like a boxer who is hitting something—not just the air. I treat my body hard and make it my slave so that I myself will not be disqualified after I have preached to others."* (1 Corinthians 9:24-17 NCV)

I don't know what it looked like to Paul, but I thought it might be helpful to you if in this chapter I would write about some of my own wrestling experiences.

Big revelation: the people in front of my eyes!

It sounds pretty funny now, looking back on it, but there actually came a day in my late 30's that all of a sudden I heard myself voice a very clear and profound revelation that my newly purified vision was forced to recon with: I said aloud to God: "Oh no—every woman has breasts—*two of them!!*" You have to laugh. But only for a moment.

What had happened is that sin had played such a role in infecting my young developing mind that when it came to encountering people of the opposite sex, I had, since age 12 or so, primarily noticed breasts (as a sexual object), and had been almost entirely unaware of the women behind them. Then at 38, as God was healing my soul/body/mind/sexuality, He was freeing my eyes to notice the profound value of all individuals. This revaluation of the personal importance of every female was a bit hard for me to follow, as I had trained my eyes—or the devil had trained my eyes—for the hunt that would satisfy dark desire; for more than 25 years, with my physical eyes and all the brain-based hardware/software/wiring that was engaged in pornographic intercourse, I had been chasing after breasts as somehow directly connected to my own personal utopia. These decades of darkness-orchestrated and hell-infused training took some undoing.

I want people who have never really struggled with this issue to at least attempt to try and understand my condition, as best as possible. We must ask God for the compassion that best echoes His heart for the lost. Perhaps a little parable will help with that endeavor. Imagine a 38-year old shark who somehow got the new revelation that he was being called to give up being a meat-eater. No matter how deeply the brain says "YES" to the transformative invitation, there is still the fact that for 38 years, that shark could smell blood, underwater, at the verified rate of 1 part per 25 million, that is, a third of a mile away in the open ocean. There is yet the fact that his eyes can still catch a flash of light glistening off a fish's scales, still be drawn to the sound of a fish in distress. If the shark is to truly become a vegan, he has a lot of reprogramming to do. And so did I. I basically had to set out to become a vegan shark.

A part of that process came to me as God was subtly pointing out that I had missed the value of so many people by only ever noticing their breasts, only ever quantifying the value of their anatomy, and only then if they were significantly attractive.

That I had lived like that for so long is still a horribly sad thought to me, and still brings tears to me eyes; it must appall and offend many who read of it here. I cannot help but wonder what it would have been like for me to never have been so impacted by darkness, to have my sexuality have escaped such plundering and hijacking. But again, it is into the darkness that Jesus Himself goes fishing, always for men such as I. He came for the lost. This is just another angle in which I must share with you how very lost I was. And its another reason why I love Him so much; because my lost state did not deter Him at all.

As I was being newly drawn to value all women, regardless of size or shape or age or any aspect of physical attractiveness, I suddenly realized that to do so I had to deliberately look at them, looking past the God-ordained beauty of their shape, raising my gaze to the beauty of faces, the windows to their souls which I had so long ignored. This was a new journey for me, and a long process. But it is one that has really become a joy.

Prayers of a vegan shark

Here is how it moved from being at first a torment to actually being a fun way of forcefully advancing the Kingdom of heaven. The Spirit of God brought Romans 12:21 to my attention: *"Do not be overcome by evil, but overcome evil with good."* During my first few weeks with redemption sharing my eyes, I was under a lot of stress: "Don't look at the breasts!! Don't look at the breasts!! Don't look at the breasts!!" This was the new constant chatter in the admin center of my brain. I was determined to walk out my repentance and not return to objectifying women. But I was also still fascinated by the God-designed beauty of the breast. In this vicious strain of trying not to notice what I was so accustomed to being aware of, I finally heard the Holy Spirit use this verse to point out that satan still was winning; he still had me totally focused on sin, and not engaged at all in worship. And it was because I was focusing only on the first part of the verse above: when all I was thinking was "Don't look at the breasts!", I was focusing on not being "overcome by evil". And it was not working!!

God invited me to take it a step further; instead of my just not being overcome by evil, He invited me to overcome evil with good. Hmmm, I pondered: "How could I do that?" *"Maybe by not ignoring the very femininity you are so dead-set on ignoring; Jeffrey, you are not going to be able to ignore it. Stop trying to. Find a way instead to use your heightened awareness of females as a very part of the process of overcoming evil with good!"* This literal interactive dialogue took only seconds; then suddenly an idea came, birthed from another scripture.

The words of Joel 2:28-29 came to me, that in the last days *" . . . I will pour out my spirit on all flesh. Your sons and your daughters shall prophesy, your old men shall dream dreams, your young men shall see visions. And also on My menservants and on My maidservants I will pour out My Spirit in those days."*

In the moment that this verse came to me, a bullet-proof strategy formed in my heart and was immediately implemented, with great and lasting success. From then on, I continued to be very aware of females. But as soon as I became aware that my attention was being unavoidably flagged by female anatomy on my visual horizon, I began to overcome evil with good by launching into the offensive, and praying with great zeal and faith:

"Dear Holy Spirit: Your promise is that in these days, You would pour out Your spirit on all flesh! I have just been made aware of a person that I might otherwise have walked past, except that their female figure caught my eye! Thank You, dear God—thank You for this woman in front of me. Thank You for drawing my attention to her. I now ask You to pour out Your Holy Spirit over her life. In keeping with Your promise, I call forth her inheritance—dreams from You, visions from heaven, the Spirit of prophecy poured over her!" Arm in arm with the very real and present Holy Spirit, empowered and unafraid, with holy vision and deep, real love flowing from me toward a woman I would likely never see again, I would continue on in intercession.

As I did so, with woman after woman I would find myself aware of, I really began to change. I wasn't perfect at it; at times I was very humbled by how long it took me to shift from anatomy awareness to praying for another bearer of God's image. But soon, I was not only noticing pretty women; I was noticing homely women, ugly women, sickly women. I was noticing classy, well kept women; I was noticing barely clothed, mistreated women. I was noticing the young and I was noticing the old. For the first time I was seeing both women with high standards as well as women with no standards, women of light and women marked by darkness.

Suddenly a whole realm of humanity I had formerly overlooked became visible to me. (How patient God was with me during this upgrade to my operating systems!) Soon, enjoying the company and excitement of the Holy Spirit, I was earnestly praying for them all.

And then, I noticed how many of them had men beside them, men I'd never noticed, men I'd never valued, men whose inheritance was promised and prophesied about in the words of Joel as well! So I started passionately praying with the Holy Spirit for the men too. And as I did so, at first admittedly as an act of war, I soon found my heart filling with a love I'd never known, praying for people everywhere as an act of sincere love and honest, holy compassion. God had used this breast-awareness issue to launch me into housing a great infusion of His heart; He had used it to engage me in love-based intercession. This is a profound strategy for turning the tables on lust.

Made to stare at beauty?

Here is another sacred contemplation. In this new journey, I began to see that perhaps in reality I really am created to gaze. Maybe it was not the gazing, the staring, the fascination with beauty that was wrong for the first decades of my being sexually active; maybe it was instead that my inner machinery of beauty location and awareness was aimed in the wrong direction. Is it possible that in fact we are all truly made to stare, transfixed, at *Something*? I began to explore this possibility.

I soon came across a text in scripture that became like a new, meditative perfume in my spirit. Under the inspiration of the Holy Spirit, King David writes of the perfect, sacred priority he discovered:

"One thing I ask from the Lord, this only do I seek: that I may dwell in the house of the Lord all the days of my life, ***to gaze on the beauty of the Lord*** *and to seek him in his temple."* (Psalm 27:4 NIV)

Strongs Concordance tells me that the Hebrew word used here is the word, *Chazah*, which means: "to gaze at; mentally, to perceive, contemplate (with pleasure); specifically, to have a vision of:--behold, look, prophesy, provide, see." Hmmm. Those words could have been used to describe the former use of my eyes in hunting beauty, noticing anatomy. I wondered if the Spirit of God was indicating my eyes were made for somehow gazing in a new direction. And if so, what would that new direction be? Was I to find a way to "gaze at God", to somehow stare at Him, captivated as I had been captivated before by lesser things? Was I to "visually contemplate" Him, perhaps even "with pleasure"?

As I began to mull this over in my mind (over the course of weeks and months and then years) some valuable rabbit trails have been introduced into my search for truth. One of them has to do with nudity itself.

The Eden behind vs the Eden ahead

In the creation account, the writer mentions that Adam and Eve *"were both naked, the man and his wife, and were not ashamed"*(Genesis 2:25). After their choice to turn against God and eat the forbidden fruit, suddenly— immediately in fact— an interesting change took place: *"(Eve) took of its fruit and ate. She also gave to her husband with her, and he ate. Then the eyes of both of them were opened, and they knew that they were naked"* (see Genesis 3:6-7). Somehow an awareness of nudity was a primary impact of the fall. This, in and of itself, deserves sacred meditation. But what you find in the English is not really the whole story.

In the English bible translations, the words "naked" used in both of the above texts are one and the same. But not so in the original. In the Hebrew, Gen. 2:25 states that the man and his wife were both *naked*—that is, *without clothing*— and yet were unashamed. But the word, *naked*, used in chapter 3:7 is a different word, and it indicates *being uncovered, having an acute awareness of danger/ vulnerability.* I am not the best one to debate the implications of these subtle differences here, but I found in this discovery that perhaps my/our hunger for gazing on nudity (at least as men) is somehow a primal awareness that there was a time that nudity was safe, a time when nudity was a primary indication that all was well and there was nothing threatening in the whole wide world. In this sense, nudity seems a possible symbol for all of Eden. It is perhaps, in one sense, representing all that was lost. Maybe we hunger for such raw beauty now because we are somehow hoping for Eden's return, hoping in fact to force our way back into the place where all that mattered was that in spite of being completely unclothed, we were also completely safe and perfectly well.

Armed with this thought, I find the draw to stare at pornography has lost its potency. In fact, I think it had been stealing power from this narrative, knowingly trying to offer me an Edenic escape, trying to slip me between the flashing swords of the angels that guard forever the entrance to the once-open gardens where shameless nudity was the rule. I know better now. Porn tries to make me look *back* to an Eden I can never attain. But God calls my vision *forward* to an Eden yet ahead of me, an Eden that, by faith, I can even now choose to stare toward, and find comfort in knowing that one day I will in fact dwell in a new heaven and earth, a place where any threat tied to vulnerability will forever be a thing of the past.

The hollowed ground of nudity

Another rabbit trail: I started noting how nudity was handled in other scriptures in a very different manner than in today's western society. A particularly odd story is recorded in Genesis 9:21-23. It is the record of the post-flood life of Noah and his sons. It tells of the day that Noah made wine from his vineyards, *". . . drank of the wine and was drunk, and became uncovered in his tent. And Ham, the father of Canaan, saw the nakedness of his father, and told his two brothers outside. But Shem and Japheth took a garment, laid it on both their shoulders, and went backward and covered the nakedness of their drunken father. Their faces were turned away, and they did not see their father's nakedness."* The text goes on to record how Noah responded: he blessed Shem and Japheth; but he cursed Ham's son.

In my pondering of a new way to look at nudity, I found this peculiar text to be very important. I cannot imagine finding two young brothers anywhere in the West who would have considered nakedness so sacred that they would lay a garment over their shoulders and walk backwards to where their drunken father lay unclothed, and in so doing, cover him up. I felt as I pondered this text that the Holy Spirit was pointing out that we of the 21st century West have lost track of how sacred nakedness is. Nudity is not funny, and is not to be taken lightly.

Along these lines, two texts related to modesty of the priests in the Old Testament Tabernacle system struck me as well. The issues of covering the dignity of human nakedness is important enough that Jehovah instructed Moses to have special linen underwear made specifically for the priests, *" . . . to cover their nakedness"* (See Exodus 28:42-43). And even with such special precautionary garments, a formal, lasting regulation was put in place to ensure that not even the slightest indecent exposure ever took place near the altar: *"And if you make Me an altar of stone, you shall not . . . go up by steps to My altar, that your nakedness may not be exposed on it'* (see Exodus 20:25-26).

Nudity seems to have a dignity about it that was not intended to be lost, stolen, or thoughtlessly, illegitimately shared. The scriptures propose the idea that nudity should be protected, preserved, highly esteemed. It turns out that modesty is important to God. So it has become important to me.

Perhaps especially because we are outside of the garden, I feel the Holy Spirit calling us men to see nudity as something hallowed, inviolable. For me, once I entered into these considerations, it was impossible to consider going back to enjoying porn; for I was suddenly aware of the predatory aspect of it in a way I had not previously been able to see. Instead of taking from people (by using porn), I was hearing a high call to find ways to protect people who, for one reason or other, are in various stages of being uncovered.

Covering my sisters

We live today in a culture that has largely lost track of the dignity of human nakedness. The wearing of apparel that leaves so much of the female body exposed is now the norm, as is the wearing of apparel that even when it covers the body, leaves much of it very tightly outlined. It is hard to believe that in just a few short years it has became so fashionable and commonplace in the West for women to wear spandex tights as if they were an outer garment. Exposure to such lack of modesty is now entirely unavoidable to the eyes of us all.

The almost constant barrage of skin and shape used to overwhelm my shark-like sensory mechanisms, but now, right in the middle of the fray, the Holy Spirit has counseled me into a call to provide covering: when we (He and I) encounter someone who is unclothed— that is, dressed with impropriety—I break into prayer with Him, asking God to take special note of this particular sister in front of me, asking Him to become a shepherd to her, to cover her in His extensive mercy, to forgive her ignorance of her own value and treasure, and to wrap her in His garments of salvation. I used to steal pleasure from underclothed individuals; now, every exposed woman who catches my eye becomes the target of sacred compassion, as the Holy Spirit and I unleash the River of Life that flows from us. It is as if He and I throw a garment over our shoulders and walk backward to cover the nakedness of the many sisters I run into that are not even aware of their own nakedness, are not even aware of their own dignity, or the gift and God-ordained power of their own beauty. And I know that in my being deliberate about providing such cover, I am not only releasing a very real blessing to these ladies, but am inviting a very real blessing to cover myself as well.

I close this chapter with a powerful little poem you might enlist in your own Holy War. In writing to Timothy, the apostle Paul instructed that he should interact with older women as if each of them were his mom, and with younger women as if each of them were his sister, all with absolute purity (1 Timothy 5:2). I have turned that excellent and liberating instruction into a simple poem that is a framework for my considerations of all women, especially the under-modest: ***"My sister, my mother, because of my Brother."*** That simple poem reminds me that the vulnerable female in front of me is not a target for lust, but is someone who falls into one of two categories: she is either a mother or a sister of mine. If her physical appearance reveals that she's in need, then what she needs me to be is a godly son, or a godly brother.

Because of my having been adopted into the family of God in which Jesus Himself is my elder brother, I can think about her from the standpoint of me being a sacred protector for the female family members I encounter.

Chapter 11 Psalm 23: a Table for Two

After 25 years of international ministry without a home base, my wife and I have been building a log home as a prayer retreat in the remote mountains of Montana. In describing the setting to people, I often use the words that came to me as the sun painted the early morning with the promises of heaven across the white tipped mountains that stab into the sky a mile away, and a mile higher than our property: I call it *Traumatically Beautiful.* I found those words in my mouth after waiting for months to get used to the tremendous landscape, with its sky-scraping evergreens and towering Rocky Mountains, its rushing rivers and glacial lakes, its pristine wildlife and overall sense of being powerfully wild and untamable. It is both traumatizing in its potential danger and its breathtaking beauty.

Sexuality is a bit like that. At least for me. Given my past, there have been times that it has been deeply traumatic for me. And if I am honest, totally aside from any aspect of darkness, I still find nudity traumatic in its very depth of beauty. My coming to peace with God and with my sexuality did not necessarily erase the traumatic side of sex. But it made it something I am *no longer afraid* of; that is, I found that it is now something whose power no longer threatens to *hurt* me. The very power of sexual beauty is still more than I know how to take in; but I'm ok with that now. I know it comes from a very *good* place, from the very drawing table of God. I now fully believe that the beauty I see in my wife is but an echo of the beyond-imagining beauty of the God whose image she is made in.

In a similar way to what's happened in me, I want to disempower the ability of sex to threaten you.

Let me come at this from yet another angle: In C.S.Lewis' wonderful work, the Lion, the Witch, and the Wardrobe, a conversation takes place between Susan (one of several heroes in the tale) and a talking Beaver (also a principle good guy) about their being on the way to meet up with Aslan (the Christ figure in the story). Mr. Beaver says to Susan at one point: "*Aslan* is a *lion- the* Lion, the *great* Lion!" "Ooh" said Susan. "I'd thought he was a man. Is he-quite safe? I shall feel rather nervous about meeting a lion!"..."Safe?" said Mr. Beaver ..."Who said anything about safe? 'Course he isn't safe! But he's good."

I can't quite find the words to convey what I sense the Spirit is saying to me, but the long and short of it is that I have come to a place of knowing that sex and nudity are similarly not "safe"—that is, not entirely predictable, or tame—but they are good! And that sacred knowing—their being firmly anchored to the goodness of God—has led me away from an over-fascination with them, and into an appropriately breath-taken, Holy Spirit-accompanied fascination with them instead.

Repentance anchor in the Shepherd's Psalm

Let's pull our hunting boots on and head down another related rabbit trail, examining along the way an additional sacred strategy: that of delayed gratification. You must have figured out reading my earlier chapters that my cycle of sin really had a demand for immediate gratification behind the steering wheel of my conscience. Since my major turn around in 2000, that has had to change. A part of that (as I touched on briefly in an earlier chapter) came from the beautiful psalm I suspect we are all very familiar with, Psalm 23. Did you ever consider that this Psalm many of us have learned as children might have anything to do with sexual purity?

The very first verse (and the whole of the psalm as well) has become for me a foundational truth that every single day of my life is built on. It's safe to say that all my repentance is anchored to it in an ongoing fashion. Let's take a look together at the empowering truths of Psalm 23:1:

"The Lord is my shepherd, I lack nothing." NIV

"The LORD is my shepherd; I have all that I need." NLT

"The LORD is my shepherd; I have what I need." CSB

As revolutionary as that simple sentence is, it is the second phrase of the verse that really has had a significant impact on my actions, on my sanctity. Specifically, it is BECAUSE the Lord is my shepherd that:

"I will never be in need." CEV

"there is nothing I lack." HCSB

"I lack nothing." NHEB

Personally, I love how it is stated, in an emphatic manner, by the NKJV:

> "The Lord is my shepherd; ***I shall not want***."

This one sentence has within it an entire strategy for pulling the plug on the stronghold behind the mask of sexual deviance.

Let's stop long enough and again, honestly ask the Spirit of Truth to help us think through the following paragraph. With His help, consider with me for a moment: what is going on when you decide that you are going to engage in pornographic intercourse, regardless of the fact that you claim to be a follower of Jesus Christ? (I know I've asked this question already in this book, but let's approach it specifically in light of Psalm 23:1.) What are you really saying in such a deliberate act? I suggest you are saying:

- *You will walk by sight, not by faith*.
- *No matter how well the Lord provides, He does not provide enough*.

Look yourself in the mirror and be man enough to finally admit that when you choose porn, you are actually aligning yourself—chaining yourself in fact— to an alternate reality, that:

- *satan is better at taking care of your needs than God!*

That is what you are really saying when you take his invitation and turn away from all God has promised you. *And that lie must be uprooted and replaced with Truth.*

Satan's core question: can God really provide?

Wake up, men: satan only ever tries to do the same trick on you that he did at the Beginning. He sneaks into your garden the same as he did in ancient Eden. He says the same line to you, asks you the same question as he did

Adam and Eve: *"Did God really say . . ?"* In our case, he asks: *"Can God really satisfy?"* In asking you this question, he draws attention to your own "rights" as part of the equation, over-exaggerating their place, and in doing so he is at the same time attacking your trust in God, attacking God's reputation, suggesting an alternative, an end to faith. In the face of such strong and effective propaganda, when we give in to his invitation to trade the promise of God's *eventual* care for the immediate gratification pornographic intercourse offers, *we are agreeing with satan's opinion of God*. And in an equally tragic mistake, *we are agreeing with satan's opinion of ourselves.* Satan is telling us God can't provide —not really, not for the deepest, most complex needs that perhaps we don't even have words for. It is as if he is telling us to redefine ourselves primarily with the overarching statement: ***I am in need***, in need beyond God's capacity to satisfy! When we let that statement become of primary importance, our character orbits an enthroned deceiver.

In the face of such blatant lies, you and I must rouse ourselves from darkness-induced slumber, and decide instead to declare this game-changing truth: that THE LORD ***IS*** MY SHEPHERD; AND THEREFORE, ***I SHALL NOT WANT!!*** The Lord IS my Shepherd, and therefore, ***I SHALL NOT BE DEFINED BY NEED!*** This is a promise-backed primary strategy in this Holy War: it is my chief declaration as I resist the devil. And when I make use of it, he flees from me (see James 4:7). This is an effective strategy that has played a significant part in my establishing myself in freedom; it can be a part of your getting out of jail free as well.

I'll be ok, thank you very much

But what does it mean, *"I shall not want?"* By making such a declaration, even should the devil flee, what happens to me, to my needs? Do they disappear? Do they go away? Are they suddenly canceled out "by faith"? Am I suddenly no longer attracted to illicit nudity? Contrary to what I'd heard from the radio preacher in Idaho, I think the honest answers have to be "no."

Forgive the abrupt redirect, but let me turn the focus of this around to you. If you are to ever walk away from your having been successfully labeled by the lie of bondage and enslaved again to darkness, you must decide if the immediacy you have been serving is worth your soul and all you hold dear. If you decide that it's not, then the only way forward out of the entangling sin is for you to begin to believe in the value of delaying the gratification of your deepest needs. My brothers, Satan is going to keep showing up at our doors, pretending to care about us, trying to help us attend to the care of our needs, as soon as possible. You have to tell him that regardless of the legitimacy of your needs, you are not going to look to his provision to see them met! Period! At times, you and I have to choose even to have our needs remain unmet, rather than have them met by satan and his schemes. End of story. End of compromise.

Of course what is really underway is an arrest of what we are calling “need”, followed by a careful, Spirit-of-God assisted inquiry into the legitimacy of that need. Careful, mature, inspired introspection will reveal that at its core, the need that must be met is a very legitimate need for intimacy, a call to be acknowledged and embraced by another. You and I were made for that and that’s ok! In fact, it’s an inseparable part of what the good design of us includes! For the one used to pornographic intimacy, it may sound ludicrous to consider that such deep, strident, pressing need might be met in any of several legitimate manners: for example, in deliberately engaging the Presence of God in true and deep worship, in interactive prayer, or of course in healthy, sacred relationship with a godly woman. But my point here is that even if there appears no option for the meeting of your deep cry for intimacy other than either engaging in pornographic intimacy or somehow delaying gratification of your deep needs until your Shepherd somehow, someday meets them out of His supernatural capacity to do so, then I must call you to the latter: I must call you to engage your own free will to shout down your needs and command yourself to line up behind the Truth that within the full spectrum of God's capacity to shepherd you, *your needs shall be covered!* And until they are, even if all you have to go by are the words of Psalm 23:1, the resounding truth in them must be enough to slay the hunger of self. He is my shepherd and therefore, I am going to be ok, thank you very much!

Die this way: the call to definitive denial

This hugely important part of the strategy to overcome temptation is called "self-denial" and it is a defining part of what it means to be a Christian.

" . . . Jesus called the crowd and his followers to him. He said, 'Any of you who want to be my follower must stop thinking about yourself and what you want. You must be willing to carry the cross that is given to you for following me.'" (Mark 8:34 ERV).

Paul unpacks the idea in these powerful verses: "*So do you think we should continue sinning so that God will give us more and more grace?* **2** *Of course not! Our old sinful life ended. It's dead. So how can we continue living in sin?*
3 *Did you forget that all of us became part of Christ Jesus when we were baptized? In our baptism we shared in his death.* **4** *So when we were baptized, we were buried with*

Christ and took part in his death. And just as Christ was
raised from death by the wonderful power of the Father, so
we can now live a new life. **5** *Christ died, and we have*
been joined with him by dying too. So we will also be
joined with him by rising from death as he did. **6** *We know*
that our old life was put to death on the cross with Christ.
This happened so that our sinful selves would have no
power over us. Then we would not be slaves to sin.
7 *Anyone who has died is made free from sin's*
control." (Romans 6: 1-7 ERV)

The New International makes the core command of this strategy clear: *"Count yourselves dead to sin, but alive to God."* The New Living Translation says it like this: *". . . consider yourselves dead to the power of sin and alive to God through Christ Jesus."* The Greek word for "count" yourselves, or "consider" yourselves, means "to take an inventory." When the devil shows up at our door and says to us, "Hey, I've got something for you that is too beautiful and powerful for you to say 'no' to!", we need to step back, take an inventory, and remember: *We have already died to sin! We are, presently, already dead to sin! Sin no longer has dominion over us!* Paul writes it in another form a few verses later: "Sin shall no longer be our master!"

These foundational choices and declarations must rise from the deepest part of who we are and come out of

our mouths to overturn the tables on the liar who tries to draw us back into darkness. This action on our part is what Paul calls "the renewing of our minds" and its how we can avoid continuing to conform to our old way of thinking and acting (see Romans 12:2).

Perhaps all of that sounds to you like an intellectual game, like mental gymnastics. But there is so much more to this discipline than meets the eye—at least for now. Which brings up another strategic rabbit trail: the delay of gratification.

Yep: I really mean He can meet ALL my needs

When I turn around and look darkness in the face and declare that I will no longer be defined by need (for comfort, or for beauty, for union, etc.) I am choosing to put off the meeting of those legitimate needs until a later date. I am not somehow so spiritual that sex no longer is of interest to me. I am not saying my needs are suddenly non-existent or that they are invalid. I am saying that if my needs cannot be legitimately met now, I am deliberately choosing to look to the meeting of them to some distant time and place, both of which are entirely in God's hands. I am choosing to place myself in the arms of God, putting all my eggs in one basket. I am declaring, as an act of Holy War on delusion, that my God shall supply *all my needs*, according to His own treasure chest of riches, embodied in the person of Christ Jesus. (Philippines 4:19)

This is faith at its core definition. *"Without faith no one can please God. Whoever comes to God must believe that He is real and that He rewards those who sincerely try to find him."* (Hebrews 11:6 EVR) God is real! And He does, for sure, reward those who sincerely try to find Him. This strategy for successfully saying "no" to sin has at its foundation that unshakable truth that there is a God, unseen for now, who will some day reward those who choose to believe Him now. *"Blessed are those," He said, "who have not seen, and still believe."* (see John 20:29)

Elsewhere, the psalmist promises again the Good Shepherd's capacity to meet our needs: *"Our Lord and our God, You are like the sun and also like a shield. You treat us with kindness and with honor, never denying any good thing to those who live right."* (Psalm 84:11 CEV)

The Lord will literally withhold no good thing from those who do what is right. Is that an amazing statement or what?! Think of it: there is nothing good that you can desire that God in heaven is wringing His hands about because He is not sure how to answer your longing. There is nothing that all of hell and mankind can create here on earth that there in heaven the Creator is wishing He had thought of first!

Keep the facts straight in your hearts and minds, and in your actions: SATAN IS NOT A CREATOR. HE IS NOT A PROVIDER. HE IS NOT CAPABLE OF MAKING YOU HAPPY! So stop screwing around with his ideas, all of which are only subtle twists of the good and perfect gifts that come down to us from the Father of lights, in whom there is no hidden darkness, no hidden small print, no disclaimers (see James 1:17). Satan's temptations only work because they are perversions of the excellent designs of heaven. James implores us with straight talk: *"You people are not faithful to God! You should know that loving what the world has is the same as hating God. So anyone who wants to be friends with this evil world becomes God's enemy.* ***5*** *Do you think the Scriptures mean nothing? The Scriptures say, "The Spirit God made to live in us* ***wants us only for Himself."*** (James 4:4-5 EVR)

Listen men: I am not interested in whether or not you are a Christian *philosophically*. You are being called now to reach beyond intellectual Christianity, beyond mental assent. Your scars from wearing the chains of this sin are requiring you to step up your faith to a new level. NOW.

Dining with Jesus while the devil watches

Once I recognized the powerful darkness that was a significant part of my own sin cycle—that is, once I realized there was a dark, supernatural personality that was using porn to hunt me down—I started to ask God to take the darkness away. I was surprised when He said to me that He would not. Instead, He pointed me to Psalm 23:5: which says that He actually prepares a meal for He and I to eat together.

That in itself is tremendously profound. It paints for me a picture of a reserved table for two—white linens, roses in a crystal vase on a candle-lit table, fine china, silver flatware, etc., etc. That in itself can transport me, to think of the God of the Universe preparing such a feast for just He and I. But that is only part of the story.

The verse goes on to say that the Good Shepherd does so *in the very presence of my enemies!* It says that while they look on, He not only dines with me, but anoints my head with oil, while His bounty overflows my place-setting. This is awesome!! It's intimate. It's beautiful. And it silences the howls of the dark.

Here's the point that has become an ongoing aspect of my victory: God doesn't kick the devil out of my life; He makes the devil watch while Jesus Himself cares for me. The devil has to personally witness the Lord, shepherding me into a place of all my needs being met. Paul writes of it in this way: *"Having disarmed principalities and powers, He made a public spectacle of them, triumphing over them . . ."* (Colossians 2:15 NKJV). That romantic table for two that Jesus prepared for me? It's surrounded by the silenced dogs of hell, who are forced to look on, tails between their legs, while Jesus wraps me in a public display of affection. Now THAT'S sacred intimacy! THAT'S a kiss to build a dream on! That's a shameless and still safe vulnerability and the seal of Perfect Love.

For twenty one years now, I have chosen that kiss over lesser loves, that "heaven, in the here and now." Even when at times I have to recreate Psalm 23 in my own sanctified imagination, I am solidly anchored in the reality that in some timeless place, God will both meet, and has already met, all my needs! That means that there are times now when I walk in pain, with a limp, or a groan in my step, because I am choosing not to medicate myself any longer with old poisons. Even if I am in pain, I am waiting for my beloved, and at the same time, am by faith experiencing His embrace even in my times of need. And if I can do that successfully, you can to. I promise you.

Chapter 12 The Beauty Beyond

This is by far the shortest chapter in this book. But there is a lot to contemplate in its subject, so I wanted this rabbit trail to have its own sacred, wide open space. I want to share with you here an important revelation that came to me as I started to re-engage with my wife, post-repentance, that is, after making my major turn around.

It was an entirely new experience for me to become one with her (sexually) while also now practicing the constant presence of God being with me; we'd be making love and I'd be deliberately reminding myself/calming my inner man (in the face of the equilibrium-bursting passion that used to signal my entering into dangerous territory during my years of misusing my sexuality) that I am not alone, that God is presently with me, even in this, even in the midst of the breathtaking wonder of sexuality and ecstasy, and the new territory of undarkened delight/desire.

At first I thought God might step away for a few minutes and leave my wife and I to ourselves; but I found that was really not His intention either. He is a gentleman, but He is also truly with us 24/7, and I sensed He wanted in some real way to be with us not just by default, but as an acknowledged and welcome contributor to our sacred communion.

I recently heard a podcast of a outspoken Christian leader and a woman, a former editor of Christianity Today, speaking about the Christian sexual experience and the book she'd just written about it. I was surprised to hear her say: "I learned certain stories from having had premarital sex all through college and in my early twenties. I learned that what's exciting and erotic about sex is this newness, and this sort of uncertainty; and that is something I am having to work to unlearn in my marriage, because of course, what's wonderful about married sex is the *ordinariness*—its not the uncertainty. But I am, if you will, having to learn that fidelity is sexy, that the ordinary can be sexy." She went on to say: "Maybe the best kind of sex is actually the most ordinary, habitual kind of sex . . . It is the appreciation of that ordinariness that I think our culture of premarital sex unfits us for, and . . . its what I suspect a lot of us are having to learn." (To hear the complete talk she gave, see Lauren Winner: What is Sex? The Naked Truth About the Facts of Life)

While I understand and am honestly in support of much of what she is trying to say, I must also interject that there is so much more, so much that is truly extraordinary about sacred sex that perhaps she has not yet tasted of. The sex that my freedom from years of impurity opened up to me is anything but ordinary or routine or habitual. What's wonderful about married sacred sex, I can say, is that it can be the truly extraordinary in a way no darkness can ever come close to replicating! I have found that sacred sex can be supernatural, in a way no other sexual union can.

I may be wrong, but perhaps when this speaker makes love, she and her husband make love "on earth", so to speak, as finite humans, as "naturals" if I may use the term. Not that that's wrong, but its so *not* the end of the road. I may sound delusional, and I'm sure my view is certainly uncommon, but now, when my wife and I come together, we somehow make love, as it were, "in heaven" rather then on earth; our union somehow occurs in connection to our being "seated with Christ in heavenly places". It has a transcendent spiritual aspect to it—as if it takes place in eternity. Honestly.

And its not just the two of us involved: God meets with us, by His Spirit, in this deepest interaction. Our intercourse is anything but routine, anything but "ordinary", or "habitual". It is always transcendent. Always new. Always tremendously different and transportive. This is because it is now ALWAYS something very Spiritual, always super-natural, always intertwined with the beauty beyond.

Chapter 13 Sex and the End of Time

A fuller understanding of what's really going on with sex in 21st century Western culture requires a look at biblical prophecy, specifically prophecy about the end of times.

"Woah," you may be thinking, wondering if I am about to go all apocalyptic. Here's the deal: I'm guessing that if you are someone still struggling with pornographic interaction, this is going to take some courage for you to even contemplate seriously, because of your perspective being anchored in the immediacy of your own passions. But Peter writes about this specific difficulty infecting society in the last days, as he writes: *"Above all, you must understand that in the last days scoffers will come, scoffing and following their own evil desires. They will say, 'Where is this "coming" he promised? . . .' "*
(2 Peter 3:3,4a NIV)

" . . . *scoffers will come* . . ." Admittedly, the word, *scoffer*, is seldom (if ever) used today and therefore invites definition. In the Greek, the word describes someone who primarily likes to make light of things, subjects that should otherwise be taken seriously. Scriptures warn us: you and

I must understand that in the last days, scoffers will scoff! That is: *people who enjoy making light of everything out there will be busy making fun of serious issues during the end of time.* They will especially make fun of those who are pointing to the return of the Lord and the end of temporal life as we know it. Peter's letter links the inappropriate timing of their mocking actions to this: that they are living according to their own passions! Several other translations say that last phrase of verse 3 this way, just to make sure you catch what is going on: at the end of the ages, scoffers will be making light of things, as they are "walking after their own lusts!"

It is unlikely that someone really devoted to his own lusts —like Joe Christian Westerner who keeps fiddling around with porn even though he is continuing to think of himself as a believer—is going to be serious about end-times prophecy. Instead, he will expect that (and act as if) things are likely to keep going on and on and on with no end in sight. But he will be wrong in this assumption. And therefore, ironically, the joke will tragically be on him. So before we go any further, dear reader, please take a moment and ask the Holy Spirit to help you understand the truth and severity of what I am about to share with you in this chapter. May the Truth cut through any mental fog, cut through any mocking spirit, that would otherwise color our understanding of the times we are in and what the Spirit of God is saying to the church in this season.

In this chapter, I will be drawing on several prophetic texts, and using them to help us understand the importance of our wrestling with what is really going on with sexuality in Western culture in the unique season we are living in.

Ultimate outpouring of the Holy Spirit

Approximately 800 years or so before the birth of Jesus, the prophet Joel wrote down a statement about "the last days." It includes this amazing prophecy of a tremendous overflow, an ultimate download from heaven:

"And it shall come to pass afterward
That I will pour out My Spirit on all flesh;
Your sons and your daughters shall prophesy,
Your old men shall dream dreams,
Your young men shall see visions.
And also on My menservants and on My maidservants
I will pour out My Spirit in those days."
(Joel 2:28-29)

First, let's unravel what is meant by "afterward" in the first sentence of the above text. On the day of Pentecost 800 years after Joel was writing, the Spirit of God poured out on the new-born church of Jesus Christ. All those of the church who were gathered together in prayer and fellowship and fasting experienced an outpouring of the

Holy Spirit, an unprecedented action during which the promise of the Holy Spirit coming to live permanently inside of humans literally took place—as if they were now His physical temple.

Jesus Himself had said this was a primary reason He had to leave His disciples: *"Nevertheless I tell you the truth. It is to your advantage that I go away; for if I do not go away, the Helper will not come to you; but if I depart, I will send Him to you."* (John 16:7) His followers were actually waiting for this to occur when the day of Pentecost arrived; they were obeying His explicit instructions, for He had said to them in His last words: *"And now I will send the Holy Spirit, just as my Father promised. But stay here in the city until the Holy Spirit comes and fills you with power from heaven."* (Luke 24:49 NLT)

I will not take the time (nor could I) to fully unpack all that took place on that pivotal, supernatural day. I will however jump to the speech Peter gave to the massive crowd that gathered, passionate as they were to understand what was going on in the lives of these common men and women who suddenly were filled with the Holy Spirit and began to display supernatural transformation. Peter explained that what they were all seeing was connected to the prophecy of Joel. Peter helps us understand the timeline of Joel's words in the verbiage of his quote. Here is what it says: *"Peter, standing up with the eleven, raised his voice and said to them, 'Men of Judea and all who dwell in Jerusalem, let this be known to you, and heed my words. . . This is what was spoken by the prophet Joel:*

'And it shall come to pass in the last days, says God,
That I will pour out of My Spirit on all flesh . . ."
(from Acts 2)

Peter goes on to quote more of Joel's words. But my point here is that he defines what Joel was writing when he said "afterward, I will pour out my spirit . . ." The specific "afterward" that Joel indicates is restated by Peter as being "after days", or "at the end of days" Peter is talking about the last days or the days near the end of time.

Both Joel and Peter, under the unction of the Holy Spirit, are giving us a clear, infallible statement about the end of time: that *one of the chief things that God will be doing then is pouring out His spirit liberally on all humanity*. The liberal outpouring is such that it will include everyone, from children to the elderly, as recipients of its message. The addresses of the young will specifically be included. The outpoured prophetic message will have no class limitations: it will be as accessible to the slave as to the bank owner, the cab driver, the doctor, the homeless, custodians, accountants, presidents, prison inmates, residents of retirement centers. ***A significant mark of the end times, Joel and Peter are shouting, is that God's voice will be accessible to all, as never before!***

Unprecedented falling away

Let's look at another text about the end of time. Our last contemplation was about the great outpouring and related potential for unprecedented infilling in the last days; this text is about a great falling away.

"Now, brethren, concerning the coming of our Lord Jesus Christ and our gathering together to Him, we ask you, not to be soon shaken in mind or troubled, either by spirit or by word or by letter, as if from us, as though the day of Christ had come. Let no one deceive you by any means; for that Day will not come unless the falling away comes first, and the man of sin is revealed, the son of perdition, who opposes and exalts himself above all that is called God or that is worshiped, so that he sits as God in the temple of God, showing himself that he is God" (2 Thessalonians 2:1-4). In short, what is clear from this awesome text is that in relation to the timing of the return of the Lord at the end of time —an event referred to in scripture as "the Day of the Lord"—there will first be *"the falling away."* Other translations refer to the falling away as the apostasy or the rebellion.

In the New Testament, Jesus Himself is the first to mention such a decline among the faithful. In Matthew 24, a chapter dedicated to His discussion with His disciples about *"the signs of his return and of the end of the age,"* He says of that specific period of time, *"And many will turn away from me and betray and hate each other."* Of course in a pursuit of God that includes the full use of free will in its foundation and economy, since Eden there has always been an ebb and flow of those who follow God and then turn away. But *THE falling away* at the end of times is so significant that it is mentioned as a key marker in sensing when Christ will return: specifically right before His return, scripture indicates there will be a *substantial* falling away.

How is this possible? During a time of unprecedented access to the outpoured Spirit of God, how might there be a corresponding falling away? Let's look for the answer to that question as this chapter unfolds further.

Societal Darkness prophesied

In writing to his young pastoral student, Timothy, Paul says the following of this same period of time:

"But know this, that in the last days perilous times will come: For men will be lovers of themselves, lovers of money, boasters, proud, blasphemers, disobedient to

parents, unthankful, unholy, unloving, unforgiving, slanderers, without self-control, brutal, despisers of good, traitors, headstrong, haughty, lovers of pleasure rather than lovers of God, having a form of godliness but denying its power. And from such people turn away!"
(2 Timothy 3:1-5)

Paul continues in this letter, writing that the people of this time period will be *". . . loaded down with sins, led away by various lusts, always learning and never able to come to the knowledge of the truth."* (v.7)

That is an extraordinarily dark description of the generation of people who have more access to heavens voice than all preceding generations. What on earth is going on in the last days?

Rise of Antichrist and the spread of filth

Another Old Testament prophet, writing about the atmosphere during the last days, points to a particularly sinister element that will severely impact society. In 11:31 and 12:11 of his writings, Daniel calls this extraordinarily evil end-times element *"the Abomination that causes desolation."* Whatever this actual item is, it is something a dark political leader (the Antichrist) will set up in the temple in Jerusalem, terminating daily sacrifices (to God). The implication is that the desolation this abomination will cause will play a society-shaping role in re-routing peoples' worship and adoration, presumably to this human king or to the demonic darkness that has infused him.

This event is significant enough that it also is mentioned by Jesus as a key sign of the times to pay attention to. In Matthew 24, in answer to his disciples inquiries about when the end of the age and the time of His own return will be, Jesus says this to His students: *"Therefore when you see the abomination of desolation,' spoken of by Daniel the prophet, standing in the holy place" (whoever reads, let him understand), "then let those who are in Judea flee to the mountains."* (Matt. 24:15-16)

What is this actual "Abomination" that causes such desolation that it needs an official title in Daniel's writings? I will be honest and say that I do not know. Even scholars of eschatology (among whom I am *not* one, to be sure) are uncertain. But that doesn't mean there isn't something for us to learn here.

What does *abomination* mean? The Hebrew word indicates something that is filthy, a pollutant, something you should loathe/hate/utterly detest.

In scripture, a search with a concordance will reveal the label of *abomination* in connection to sexual sin (specifically adultery, incest, homosexuality, and bestiality —see Leviticus 18) and to societal engagement in idolatry and the related offering of children in sacrifice to idols (see 1 Kings 11:7; 2 Kings 23:13).

Filth that causes staggering ruin

Like the word, *abomination*, *desolation* is a word we use very little, so it begs definition as well. Merriam Webster Dictionary defines it as follows:

- **1** the action of desolating: the pitiful *desolation* and slaughter of World War I — D. F. Fleming
- **2 a:** grief, sadness: … he put his trembling hands to his head, and gave a wild ringing scream, the cry of *desolation.* — George Eliot
  b: loneliness
- **3:** devastation, ruin: a scene of utter *desolation*
- **4:** barren wasteland: looked out across the *desolation*

To best understand, I looked up (Merriam Webster again) the word, *desolate*, and found it meant:

- **:** devoid of inhabitants and visitors **:** deserted—a *desolate* abandoned town

- **2:** joyless, disconsolate, and sorrowful through or as if through separation from a loved one: a *desolate* widow
- **3 a:** showing the effects of abandonment and neglect **:** dilapidated: a *desolate* old house
  b: barren, lifeless: a *desolate* landscape
  c: devoid of warmth, comfort, or hope**:** *gloomy, desolate* memories

Whatever the actual Abomination Daniel is writing about is, it will apparently be the cause of extensive devastation, ruin, grief, and barrenness to society. But Daniel indicates it brings even more than the English dictionary explains. In the Aramaic that his book is written in, the word means as well *to stupefy, to amaze, to make wonder, to astonish, self-destruction.*

Strategic mesmerizing evil in the last days

My point in bringing all this up is not in any real way to attempt to identify and define *THE* Abomination or to spend significant time in speculating on its reality. In fact, what I am about to say is NOT a definition of the actual abomination or the specific desolation it will bring. What I DO feel drawn to ponder is this: a defining characteristic of the atmosphere at the end of time, is that there will be released into society something mesmerizing and horrific, something that causes both amazement—the captivating of attention—and desolation, and that such horrific devastation will be along the lines of captivating/enslaving the minds of men and women, drawing them into self-destruction through re-routing the energy of proper worship into significant societal idolatry, likely to include sexual error.

Having read through the earlier chapters of this book in your hands, can you not sense now the strategic role of pornographic intimacy— specifically through the introduction and proliferation of internet/computer based sexual intimacy —in bringing hair-raising devastation to global society in these darkening days? Although it is not THE abomination that will cause such devastation, internet pornography is, in my opinion, a pre-echo of it, being a lesser earthquake that similarly is an abomination that causes desolation.

Historic link: demons mating with humans

Hmmm. Might there be other end-times prophecies that include the coming of such darkness—specifically, idolatrous/adulterous sexual intimacy with demons? I think the answer to that question is yes. But before we look at a text that mentions such troubling *future* darkness, we need to look far back in time, looking over our shoulder all the way to the time before the flood in Genesis.

Noah lived in an extremely troubling time. Although there were likely many dark aspects of his society that drew God's attention, there is one shocking specific recorded in Genesis 6 that was THE primary concern: fallen angels were actually having sex with humans. Scripture records that fallen angels visited the earth, found themselves attracted to human females, and somehow joined themselves in sexual union. The result of their copulating with the human women was the corruption of the human species and the birth of the giants. (See Genesis 6, 1-4). Directly after reporting this astonishing condition of dark intimacy, the text goes on to report one of the saddest verses in all scripture. *"Then the Lord saw that the wickedness of man was great in the earth, and that every intent of the thoughts of his heart was only evil continually. And the Lord was sorry that He had made man on the earth, and He was grieved in His heart."* (v.5-6)

The impact of man having fallen to such a level of demonically intwined depravity is cataclysmic; the hammer falls in the very next verse:

"So the Lord said, 'I will destroy man whom I have created from the face of the earth, both man and beast, creeping thing and birds of the air, for I am sorry that I have made them.' "

To recap the situation: Dark spiritual entities had visited the earth and engaged in sexual union with human women, deliberately corrupting humanity, and actually fathering hybrid physical beings— mighty men, giants—spawning a corresponding spread of darkness that was so pervasive that it was almost completely universal; as a result, every intent of the thoughts of men's hearts became only continually evil. And the scope and effect of this deliberate corruption was not limited to humans; scripture indicates the infection brought by darkness actually corrupted the whole earth (v 11). In His perfect wisdom, God, with a broken heart, decides the judgement that is necessary to right the ship and save the world is so extensive that it requires not only the destruction of almost all human life, but also the deaths of all animate forms of life. *Only Noah and his family and the animals sent to him in the ark he builds will survive this terrific judgement and repopulate the cleansed earth.* Such is the important Old Testament account.

The flood did not come because people just progressively became more and more sinful over time and finally needed a reset: the flood came because supernatural darkness was deliberately, strategically corrupting the earth through some sort of literal copulation between earth and hell.

Now lets take a look at a related New Testament statement of Jesus. *"But as the days of Noah were, so also will the coming of the Son of Man be.* ***38*** *For as in the days before the flood, they were eating and drinking, marrying and giving in marriage, until the day that Noah entered the ark,* ***39*** *and did not know until the flood came and took them all away, so also will the coming of the Son of Man be."* (Matthew 24:37-39)

To be clear, I think Jesus primary indication in this text is that mankind, pre-flood, had no idea of the judgement that was rushing toward them until it was too late, and that in a very similar manner, in the last days, mankind will be completely oblivious to the fact of their own impending doom, as world-wide cataclysmic judgement again rushes toward them. This characteristic is mentioned in several passages, chiefly by the mention of the Lord's return as being like the coming of a thief to ones' home in the middle of the night.

I recognize that this primary lack of awareness of the serious nature of the times at hand is the chief message of what Jesus is meaning when he says, *"As it was in the days of Noah, so will the coming of the son of man be."* However, as I journeyed with the Holy Spirit's help away from the dark supernatural intimacy that *I* had been toying with, I sensed an echo in this prophecy, an echo of the demonic darkness that brought on the flood in Noah's time. Although it is purely conjecture on my part and must be understood as such, I think it is very real that in this generation, we have at our convenience suddenly a globally accessible means of sexually interacting with demons through pornographic intimacy, the like of which seems to me to be very reminiscent of the days of Noah when supernatural union between darkness and humans produced the corruption of society, tremendous mental/spiritual decline, and led directly to the destruction of almost all animate life on the planet. I do not think it will be a coincidence if the extent of such widespread pornographic intimacy with darkness does not similarly invite/require a judgement that will necessarily purify the planet again in its complete reset of all life on this planet.

Apocalyptic porn: gateway to demons

Why do I bring up several ancient prophecies in a book dealing with 21st century internet porn? I bring it up because I think in a very real sense, the devil is totally freaked out about the first prophecy we looked at in this chapter, the words of Joel chapter 2. Let me restate that: one of the keys that I feel the Holy Spirit brought to my attention as He rescued me from porn's attractive power is that the devil is very aware of Joel's prophecy of this tremendous outpouring of access to God in the end of time, and that therefore he (the devil) is doing all he can to create distraction and to contaminate the airwaves, so to speak, to corrupt as many as possible in an effort to prevent the Message from Heaven ever reaching the ears of "all flesh." Global human access to God's Voice is what is at stake here; the purity of the target of Christ's affection is the venue for such an outpouring. Hence the launch of a supernatural conflict, an all out effort to release global desolation through widespread supernatural intimacy with darkness— literally a devastation-producing outpouring of a spirit of filth and pollution— instead of the promised outpouring of the Holy Spirit.

I think its vitally important that we all wake up to the reality that porn, as a gateway to demonic intimacy, is one of the chief end times strategic weapons in the devil's hands. I propose that his concept is that if he can make society impure on a global level, perhaps God's Spirit will not pour out on all flesh. The computer that now resides in every mans' pocket offers access today to the expansive offer of 40 million pornographic websites; I suspect that such unparalleled offers of deep adultery/idolatry, joined increasingly with rapidly developing virtual reality technologies, threaten the earth with a similar darkness to the one that covered the earth in Noah's day. You and I must awaken to the call to have absolutely nothing to do such strategic contamination.

Let me inject a final serious dose of truth into this chapter's journey. James writes rather bluntly in his book: *"You people are not faithful to God! You should know that loving what the world has is the same as hating God. So anyone who wants to be friends with this evil world becomes God's enemy. Do you think the Scriptures mean nothing? The Scriptures say,* ***'The Spirit God made to live in us wants us only for himself.'*** " (James 4:4-5 ERV)

Dear reader, God is jealous for you! He wants to live inside of you! You are the temple He has chosen to dwell in. And in order for Him to do so, to safely come and share the home you live in, He passionately wants you all to Himself.

The obvious flip side of this coin is that the enemy of our souls also wants us only for himself. *Herein lie the grounds for Holy War.*

Chapter 14 Royal Invitation

*"Then the angel showed me Joshua the high priest
standing before the angel of the Lord. The Accuser, Satan,
was there at the angel's right hand, making accusations
against Joshua.* **2** *And the Lord said to Satan, 'I, the Lord,
reject your accusations, Satan. Yes, the Lord, who has
chosen Jerusalem, rebukes you. This man is like a burning
stick that has been snatched from the fire.'*

3 *"Joshua's clothing was filthy as he stood there before
the angel.* **4** *So the angel said to the others standing there,
'Take off his filthy clothes.' And turning to Joshua he said,
'See, I have taken away your sins, and now I am giving you
these fine new clothes.'*

5 *"Then I said, 'They should also place a clean turban on
his head.' So they put a clean priestly turban on his head
and dressed him in new clothes while the angel of the Lord
stood by.*

6 *"Then the angel of the Lord spoke very solemnly to Joshua and said,* **7** *'This is what the Lord of Heaven's Armies says: If you follow my ways and carefully serve me, then you will be given authority over my Temple and its courtyards. I will let you walk among these others standing here.' "* (Zechariah 3: 1-7 NLT)

As I sat down to write this chapter on holiness, immediately I felt the Holy Spirit suggest I start with this tremendous scripture from the prophet, Zechariah. It is, for me, one of the most amazing accounts of the war that takes place between the Accuser of man and the Savior/ Redeemer over the well being of a lowly sinner. Although the man in the sacred tug of war recorded here is named Joshua, the record echos so clearly to me what must have taken place in heaven as I was standing, filthy and sin-ruined, rightly accused before the Holy God, and as Heaven's Voice basically stepped in front of me to tell a mocking satan to shut up and go to hell.

This chapter, reflecting the transformation Zechariah reported above, is about some of the final steps of my supernatural reformation. Like Joshua, I had been snatched as a stick out of the fire and my accuser had been silenced and my sins forgiven; now it was time for my mind to receive a new turban, a new way of thinking, before I was ready to be really commissioned into a new way of life. That pivotal new way of thinking had to do with what it means to be holy.

Holy, as God is, or filthy loser?

At some point during this sensitive season of rebirth and paradigm shift, I had been presented with a scripture that left me troubled:

"So prepare your minds for action and exercise self-control. Put all your hope in the gracious salvation that will come to you when Jesus Christ is revealed to the world.
14 *So you must live as God's obedient children. Don't slip back into your old ways of living to satisfy your own desires. You didn't know any better then.* ***15*** *But now you must be holy in everything you do, just as God who chose you is holy.* ***16*** *For the Scriptures say, "You must be holy because I am holy."* (1 Peter 1:13-16 NLT)

The key phrase that left me uncomfortable was the closing statement: "be holy . . ." My mind kept repeating the phrase in a misquoted fashion; I kept pondering it in these words: "be holy, *as* I am holy." The burr in my saddle came from the word, "as". Although I have since tried to find a translation that I might have had access to at the time that also used this word, "as", I cannot now find it. I must suggest that it may have come from the DUV, that is, the Devil's Unauthorized Version— I honestly think the accuser was injecting this word into the text in order to discourage me. You and I must remain aware that satan is pretty good at misquoting what God says in order to trip us up (See Gen. 3: 1-5 and Matt. 4: 5-6). In the raw state of my having been freshly snatched from the fires of my sinful choices, even I could see that there was no way I could be holy *AS* God is holy, no way I could be innocent, spotless, and pristine in the same way that *He* is. With the insertion of that little word "as", this text that kept playing through my mind was translated by my heart as "BE PERFECT, just as God is perfect!!" Contemplating what felt to me to be a clear command—BE HOLY, AS I AM HOLY—that seemed impossibly unattainable, I felt depressed by the chasm between God's capacity for holiness and my own. The more my heart tried to contemplate obeying the command, the more the text began to hang over me, like a scream of accusation, until the verse sounded in my spirit like this: *"You can't be holy, like God is Holy!! Ha ha—you're so deluded—you are, and will always be, just a filthy loser!"*

It is the role of the Holy Spirit to lead us into all truth (John 16:13) and to bring comfort. And so He came to me and suggested I take a deeper look at the command that was really beginning to trouble me. He led me to look up and dig into the scripture Peter quotes above, from Leviticus:

"For I am the Lord your God. You must consecrate yourselves, and be holy, because I am holy. So do not defile yourselves . . . For I, the Lord, am the one who brought you up from the land of Egypt, that I might be your God. Therefore, you must be holy, because I am holy." (Leviticus 11: 44-45 NLT. The same is repeated in Leviticus 19:2 and 20:7)

Identified as peculiar

Having rescued the children of Israel from 400 years of enslavement in Egypt and from the collection of gods of that nation that the Israelites must have been very familiar with, Yahweh was taking the time to explain a few things to this million+ strong group of refugees. In the desert, between their former prisons and future promised land, He invested a lot of effort in introducing them to Himself: primarily they were learning that He was good, as opposed to the gods they had known before who had subjected them to endless punishment and the slaughter of their own children. They were learning that Yahweh was capable of caring for their needs, as opposed to the gods whom they had known before, who had only thrived on the very backs of the children of Israel. They were finding out that He was all powerful, as opposed to the gods they had just seen entirely trampled in Egypt. There were any number of ways in which Yahweh demonstrated that He was different than all the other gods they had known. In fact, it would be fair to say that He was making it plain to them that He was set apart from all that they knew about other gods; He was different. He was in a separate category, consecrated, dedicated. That is part of what He meant when He said to them that He was Holy.

And because He was now their god, and they His children, it followed that He was inviting them to similarly see themselves as set apart, different, consecrated, dedicated. Because He was so different, so extraordinarily set apart from all other gods, He was inviting these former slaves—the very bottom of the social ladder—to see themselves as extraordinarily different too, as peculiar, as special: to see themselves as *Holy*.

He explains this new concept in several other passages: in a fatherly talk recorded in Leviticus 10, He explains to His children that they must develop a new focus of discernment as a part of their maturing:

"You are to distinguish between the holy and the common, and between the unclean and the clean . . ." (v.10 EV)

In a passage that records the duties of the priests within society, Ezekiel writes:

"And they shall teach My people the difference between the holy and the unholy, and cause them to discern between the unclean and the clean." (Ez. 44:23)

We could actually write an entire study book on this concept, for it was at the very foundation of God's efforts to take the lowest, most trampled individuals and bring them into the revelation of their being lifted up and invited into positions of royal sonship through this invitation to holiness.

As I reflected on these and so many other similar verses, I felt the Holy Spirit's hand under my chin, as it were, lifting my face to gaze on a new consideration: the command to BE HOLY was nothing less than a truly extraordinary opportunity to leave my past behind. As this revelation began to penetrate my downtrodden heart, Holy Wind began to fill my sails, and I began to see the command in a whole new light.

Celebrating leaving the past behind

I now see that the call to holiness is nothing less than the best possible news—it is in fact a celebrational celestial invitation to a life far beyond what I might ever have found outside of God. The call and command to be holy is now to me the call to become something absolutely amazing and truly wonder-filled. Instead of hearing the accuser mockingly misquote those words to me, I now here the exuberant voice of my smiling Jesus, cheering me on with these words:

"Be transcendent, as I am transcendent!

"Be radically purposeful, as I am full of purpose!

"Be extraordinary! Be exceptional! Be phenomenal! Be remarkable! Be noteworthy!

"See yourself as uncommonly valuable, as I am uncommonly valuable!

"Think higher, HIGHER, about yourself, and about the choices set before you—in fact, come on up here, out of the trash heap you've dug through in the past, and sit down with Me in heavenly places!! I know where you came from, but I want you right up here, sitting on my throne with me. You are no longer a commoner; you are my royal son! And I am inviting you to participate in the divine nature!" (See 2 Peter 1:4 and Revelation 3:21)

I want to make it clear that I am in no way trying to lessen the call to be separated from *sin*. This chapter is certainly not a full treatise on the topic of holiness. But in my own journey to separate myself from a life dominated by sin, the Holy Spirit called me to understand that holiness is a call to so much more than just NOT doing something wrong. That old call to holiness had no power in my life, as long as I heard it from a scolding voice and had it accompanied with a wagging finger; when holiness became an invitation to all the wonder of the uncommon existence Yahweh was offering to me, I traded my sin-focused mindset for one aimed at sacred adventure and truly became something supernatural. And so, I moved from being afraid of holiness to being captivated by it and drawn to run to it! I now love the thought of being holy, of doing holy things.

Anybody can be unholy. That's easy! But I am not just anybody; I'm set apart. I'm special. I'm holy. And I make choices that demonstrate that now I no longer believe the lie that I am nothing, or that I am a loser. I am *not* a loser! I am a triumphant winner, an overcomer! And I am Holy!

"Be Holy, because I am Holy." What a delightful invitation!

Chapter 15 To Know and be Known

Matthew records some interesting information about Darkness at work inside of an individual.

"When an unclean spirit goes out of a man, he goes through dry places, seeking rest, and finds none. Then he says, 'I will return to my house from which I came.' And when he comes, he finds it empty, swept, and put in order. Then he goes and takes with him seven other spirits more wicked than himself, and they enter and dwell there; and the last state of that man is worse than the first. So shall it also be with this wicked generation."
(Matthew 12: 43-45)

I am not going to open up an extensive debate here about the mechanics of, or even the possibility of, demon possession in the life of a believer. For me its very simple to understand that ***if*** you open doors to darkness—especially if you are willfully, repeatedly making dark, sinful choices—you ***will*** open yourself up to be mentally/spiritually/psychologically influenced by darkness. But more than discuss that issue, I felt led to start this final chapter with the above text to introduce a hopeful picture of a future you may not yet have dreamed of. I have no interest in leading you to a place where you are only swept clean; I want to take you to a place where the beautiful Bridegroom, Jesus, fills the void that false intimacy was trying to fill. That is something worth cleaning house for!

As you have come along with me on the journey through this book, you witnessed my having been almost completely unaware of the reality of the supernatural, living out my life in a state of passive unbelief (in spite of my upbringing as a conservative christian). Although grossly unaware of the reality of dark supernatural entities, I never the less found myself in bed with them, literally having supernatural intercourse with darkness through the portal of pornography and masturbation. But God, with both creative consequential measures and a bold smile, stepped into that chaotic arena, warning me of my unbelief, and turning the lights on behind the charade of pornographic intercourse. And when I could see the darkness behind my choices, the Truth liberated my will and set me free, through my own choices for freedom, free from the bondage that would have eventually killed me and left my soul in the lake of fire forever.

Somewhere in that journey that took maybe a little over a year for me to go from A to Z, I was saved—truly, radically saved. I was saved from having dark supernatural intercourse, saved from having sex with the devil. That's a bit graphic to say it that way, but that is really what I was saved FROM. But what is it I was saved TO?

Sacred Supernatural Intercourse. I was saved from having supernatural intercourse with darkness, so that I might begin to live a life of supernatural intimacy with Light!

After decades of fascination with sex dominating my existence, once I was truly set free and redeemed, I was delighted to find out from scripture that I was saved so that I might become truly one—truly united, truly intimate—with God. Perhaps the wording sounds strange or not quite religious enough to our fallen minds, but they are more true than I was aware: in the truest spiritual sense, at my core, I was made for the deepest possible kiss, for truest possible intimacy with God. I was made for the Song of Solomon 1:2 kisses of the mouth of God.

Am I going too far? Let's find out by looking at the scriptures that the Holy Spirit brought to me, as my house was being cleaned out and prepared for new and sacred Romance and Resident.

I found myself puzzling one day over a text that really is very serious. It involves a parable where Jesus talks about the possibility of someone coming before Him at the end of time, someone full of expectation that they are, on the basis of their own considerably impressive religious activity, about to receive a warm welcome by the Son of God. Instead, He stuns them with these incomparably horrific words: *"Get away from me; I NEVER KNEW YOU!"* (See Mathew 7: 21-23)

This grave terminology is echoed in the parable of the ten virgins, where half the ladies show up late, yet full of expectations of a welcome, only to hear the same blistering statement from the lips of Jesus: "For sure, I'm telling you— I DON'T KNOW YOU!" (See Mathew 25: 1-11)

He doesn't know them? How could that be possible? I thought He knew everything . . . In my contemplative heart, I felt a draw to understand what this word KNOW was all about. As it related to my recent freedom from dark intimacy and to my recent embrace of the invitation to holiness, the Holy Spirit took me into the Old Testament to help me understand what I was finding in the New.

Yada: fullest possible awareness

He took me first to Genesis chapter 4. There we find these words at the start of the chapter:

"Now Adam ***knew*** *Eve his wife, and she conceived . . ."*

(v.1) Hmmm. He *knew* her, and the result was that she became pregnant: now that's some KNOWING!

That word translated as "knew" in this verse is the Hebrew word, *Yada*. The Strong's concordance has a lengthy definition that starts as follows: "to know (properly, to ascertain by seeing); used in a great variety of senses, figuratively, literally, euphemistically and inferentially (including observation, care, recognition . . .)" There is quite a bit more to the definition but the point is actually pretty simple and clear: the Hebrew definition of "know" is not very unlike our English understanding of "knowing". Simply put, *knowing* is about fullest possible awareness of, and to the Hebrew mind, there was no separation of the mental from the physical/sexual identity involved in the possible landscape of one *knowing* and *being known*. Adam ***knew*** Eve—Adam had in-depth intimate awareness of all that Eve was in her deepest most private world; the result of such an in-depth discovery was that union took place, a blurring of the boundaries of where Adam ended and where Eve began. The two became one. *Such is the end goal of knowing and being known.* Actually, not only the *end*; the result of the 'knowing" was also a *beginning* —pregnancy and childbirth flowed from the intimate interchange.

We see the same word, *Yada*, used in a different manner in Genesis 18:19. In this text, we are reading of God "knowing" the patriarch, Abraham: *"For I have* ***known*** *him, in order that he may command his children and his household after him, that they keep the way of the Lord, to do righteousness and justice, that the Lord may bring to Abraham what He has spoken to him."* Again, in the deepest core interaction—the intimacy— between God and Abraham, an exchange took place, and Abraham received and embraced aspects of the Supernatural that would not only end in him being "closer" in relationship to God, but also would produce fruit—contributing to Abraham's capacity to father supernaturally the nation that would come from his loins as a result of this "knowing."

Yada is also in the text of Exodus 33:13 *"Now therefore, I pray, if I have found grace in Your sight, show me now Your way, that I may* ***know*** *You and that I may find grace in Your sight. And consider that this nation is Your people."*

Of course, this time the speaker is Moses, and the request in his prayer is simply this: "God, I want nothing between us—I don't want there to be any secrets. I need the fullest possible awareness of all that you are; I am now fathering a nation and in order to do so well, I absolutely must *know* You most intimately."

The Prophet Daniel uses a similar word (in Aramaic) in his discussion of the end of time. In Daniel 11:32 he makes this profound statement about life during a very dark time, during which intimate connection to God will be *absolutely vital*: *" Those who do wickedly against the covenant, he* (aka, the antichrist) *shall corrupt with flattery; but the people who* ***know*** *their God shall be strong, and carry out great exploits."*

Hosea also makes mention of the crucial necessity of such intimacy, where again we hear things from God's perspective: *"My people are destroyed for lack of* ***knowledge****. Because you have rejected* ***knowledge****,*
I also will reject you from being priest for Me; Because you have forgotten the law of your God, I also will forget your children." (Hosea 4:6)

Even under the old covenant, deep intimacy with God was not an option, not extra curricular activity; it was instead God's highest goal and prerequisite for life and wellbeing in the fullest sense.

Scores of other examples of this word, *Yada*, fill the pages of the Old Testament. But the concept of the highest priority of deepest intimacy is not limited to the Hebrew.

Although written in Greek, the underlying concept in the pages of the New Testament is the same; when Jesus says to shocked followers, *"Depart from me, I never knew you!"*, He is speaking to primarily spiritually dead religious people who are trying to get in on the benefits of relationship with Him without the homework involved in true intercourse; to them He says the truth: *"Get away from me—we were never truly intimate!"*

New way to be human: 24/7 in God's arms

This is my "weltanschauung", my new world-and-life view: I fully believe that I was created for intimate interaction with the Creator of the universe, the Lover of my Soul, the Bridegroom of my spirit. This goes far beyond the fullest intellectual study of theology. This is far more than academia. This is, in fact, Divine Romance. This is real relationship on the deepest level with the triune God.

I fully believe all the time I spent in chaos and confusion and in bondage dabbling with darkness is due to the reality that satan hates God's offer of deepest loving interaction with me and is working desperately to prevent it from coming to pass. But greater is He that is in me then he that is in the world. The love of God chased after me until it found me, and rescued me from the dark embrace I mistakenly had stepped into. My search has ended—or perhaps now has only truly begun—in a life of growing supernatural intimacy with the God who has made it His expressed primary interest to get to KNOW me and have me KNOW Him in return. To this shocking and wonderful invitation, I have thrown my hands up in ecstatic surrender, and said (and say again with every new day) a resounding YES! I have closed the doors on the dead-end of false intimacy and have opened my heart to the wild, endless adventure of being kissed with the kisses of Heaven's mouth. To know Him and to be known by Him—for this I live!

But this story is really not only about me. This is OUR story. Please say that it is so!

Dear reader, I hope these personal testimony-filled pages have offered hope to you in your search for life and freedom and the inner peace and satisfaction that is only attainable in the arms of our Holy God. I pray my words have opened your heart to the reality that you, too, are being courted— both by Life and by Death— and that you too must choose to fight against intimacy with darkness with everything you have inside of you.

The great news is: Today really IS the day of salvation! Today the doors of grace are wide open! Today, nothing you could finally confess will surprise the Lover of your soul, nor diminish His offer to you of a whole new life, if you will truly, radically change your mind about the supernatural realm, about sex, about pornographic intimacy, and eternity, and the fabulous invitation to leave all our mistakes drowned beneath the holy blood of Jesus Christ, as you step into fullest freedom and the abundant life waiting for you!

Today, hear His voice, and do not harden your heart against His matchless offer of supernatural love.

I close with what is both a solemn and an effervescent invitation, written so long ago but still so relevant to the subjects discussed in these few pages:

"I call heaven and earth as witnesses today against you, that I have set before you life and death, blessing and cursing; therefore choose life, that both you and your descendants may live; that you may love the Lord your God, that you may obey His voice, and that you may cling to Him, for He is your life and the length of your days . . ." (From Deuteronomy 30:19,20)

Come out, come out, wherever you are! Let there be no more hiding from the call to truest intimacy and the wonder found only in and through His embrace. Hear and respond to this incomparable offer from your Beloved: *"Rise up my love, my fair one, and come away with me!"*

(from Song of Solomon 2)

Afterword

You and I were *made* for Intimacy! Really!

In my darkest hours, in the absence of appropriately diligent deliberate parental interaction, in the subtle neglect of my developing personhood as a child, and in the wake of the sexual exploitation that I was the target of, I had surrendered to isolation and disconnection from the society that I needed. Even though God and His answers to my problems were really never far away, I came to believe the well-positioned lie that meaningful relationship with Him was entirely beyond my reach. And I became stranded.

As such, I was an easy target for the devil, who scripture clearly says "roams around looking for someone to devour". For me, the devouring became residential as I yielded the right for him to place me into a functional solitary confinement. But those days are over now, forever!

My sincere desire is that your hearing me say that gives you tremendous hope: your extended days of duplicity and isolation and self betrayal can be behind you. And stay behind you.

Most of this book you have just read was about me awakening to the poison I had swallowed in my youth. I now know this: there is no lie that can withstand the power of the Truth. Once I knew the Truth, in the very same manner that Jesus said it would, the Truth set me free!

My life from that point on has been so tremendously different! Truth has become my reality anchor. First the change was maintainable only moment by moment, hour by hour; I literally printed out vital scriptures, declarations, and prayers (taken from Neil Anderson's life saving book, The Bondage Breaker) and carried those around with me day and night to refer to, read through, and re-declare aloud as I was literally laying new tracks of thought for my renewed mind to run on. I was zealous for my liberty and jealously guarded against the return of darkness; you must do the same, with your whole heart, mind and strength. In short, you must ***really love*** the Lord your God. In so doing you will *" . . . work out your own salvation with fear and trembling."* (From Phil. 2:12)

The Word of God is powerful and alive (see Hebrews 4:12). We live on every word that proceeds from the mouth of God (Matthew 4:4). Staying whole and holy for me has meant that I continually keep Jesus' power-embedded words always in front of me, my mind focused on His truths as if they were engraved on the inside of my eyelids. That is what escaping from my bondage to sin has required of me. I have chosen to LOVE life and to HATE any compromising choice I might otherwise make (a.k.a., *sin*). With Ephesians 4:27 as a motto—"*. . . do not give the devil a foothold*"— I make every effort to *never give him even a tiny amount of real estate on which to rebuild prison walls around me*.

Walking in holiness will require the same of you. Like the psalmist writes so plainly in Psalm 1, the only man who will be blessed is the man who delights in the law of God and meditates on it day and night; consistent health and fruitfulness can really only flow from such a happily rooted, focused life, planted firmly by the effervescent rivers of living water.

In these pages, I have tried to share with you the somewhat peculiar details of how my prison sentence came to an end, and how I got out of jail free. It is my hope that the testimony will radically inspire your shift out of darkness into the glorious, intimate, and unbreakable embrace of Jesus. I don't use the word "radical" lightly; I do pray you decide to radically, decisively bring an end to any duplicity in your life. Right now. And if that is the case — if you are finally in the process of seeing the God of peace crush satan under *your* feet—then before I close, I want to strongly encourage you as well to meditate day and night on the living word of God, and to very deliberately engage in the practice of ongoing intimacy with Him.

Here are some final tips to help with that process.

~Talk to Him. Endlessly.

Dont worry about format. Maybe don't even think of it as "prayer" right now. Just TALK to Him. He is a *person*. And He is in love with you, the sound of your voice, the appearance of your face. (See Song of Solomon). Some call this prayer; but if that is what it is, then prayer must become a way of life. As St. Paul charged us: *"Pray continually."* (1 Thess. 5:17 NIV) My paraphrase? "Don't let the conversation between you and God ever stop!"

~Read His letters to you. Listen to them on your audio devices. *"Let the message about Christ, in all its richness, fill your lives."* (Colossians 3:16a NLT). Make the effort of finding a solid Bible translation that will also reach your heart and really open you to hearing His personal voice speak in a language you respond to. (FYI: For me that meant leaving the KJV—in which I had memorized nearly 1000 verses during my years of struggle—and shifting into NIV, NLT, and then NKJV (where I spend most of my study time now), all of which were like an entirely different experience for me; their lack of formality suddenly opened my heart to hear Gods voice. It was as if the archaic tone of the KJV was a form of a religious barrier; it actually kept God at a distance from me throughout my years of duplicity. I know many for whom the KJV has not built this barrier; but such was my experience. The long and short of it is: you must find a translation that echos the truth that the scriptures are meant to be fully alive and personal to you.)

~Find a means of burying yourself in worship (in spirit and in truth), where the organic focus is on the beauty of God and His being worthy of your attention and affection. I recommend you begin a study of worship that will be ongoing and lifelong; take what you are learning from that study and put it passionately into practice. I strongly encourage your exploration of and participation in the relatively recent global awakening to the power and calling of corporate night and day worship and intercession. (See Appendix A for recommended books on this topic.)

~Just do it! Your involvement in all of these new things may seem contrived at first; it may seem fake. But remember, you are unwinding yourself from what *SEEMED* real but really was fake—intimacy with darkness. Decide in your heart that you will read/listen to the Bible, you will worship, and pray, and study and meditate on truth day and night, and use your voice to declare the truth— no matter how it feels, or doesn't feel. In time, you will find yourself falling deeply in love. As you move toward Him, you will encounter the fulfillment of the promise: "Draw near to God, and He will draw near to you." For regardless of the lies the enemy has told us, you and I were made for love!

~Find family! It turns out we were really made for family! What a great discovery that is! In 1998-99, the Word of God finally transformed my private, internal world. But the effect of it did not stop there: it also opened up a place in the Kingdom of Heaven family for me, a place that guilt and shame had previously welded shut. It is offering to do the same for you right now!

By God's design and orchestration, your new life—like mine—will eventually dovetail with others in corporate expression of Kingdom family. Be deliberate about connecting in honesty and openness with other believers. In God's time and way, He will place you in a family expression. Believe His word about this and trust Him as you wait for what that will look like: He's promised to place the lonely in family (Psalm 68:6).

This shift—from isolation, duplicity, and solitary confinement to openness and redemptive family embrace — is such a vital avenue for the flow of life that must become a part of the existence of anyone who wants to really leave the past behind and step into the fullness of life Jesus purchased for us. However, although the perfect love, endless grace, and tremendous mercy of God are, in reality, scandalously accessible, your transition from sin-stained isolation and internal solitary confinement into lasting, redemptive family embrace may be a bit more of a complex shift to see realized. If your road forward to family is not so straightforward, d*on't be put off by speed bumps or detours in the journey*: your faith is being tested and strengthened along the way. Prove to Jesus that you can be, and are, faithful, whether you are all alone for an extended period or are deeply embraced right away by healthy kingdom brothers and sisters.

~Testify! When God lets you know that it's time, tell your story. It's possible that some people may be freaked out by what you and I have been through. So what. Don't worry about it! The bottom line is: you were lost; it may have taken you a while but you finally admitted it and cried out for help. Now you are found! That's the story line. Make it yours. Be deliberate and confident and shameless about that fact that *your life is the perfect canvas for a haunted and searching world to know how truly beautiful is the Savior of the Lost and the Bridegroom of Humanity.*

So keep owning your redemptive story. Share it. When you start to do so, it may feel to you like the first time you held hands with a girlfriend in public—a bit awkward and shy and silly, while at the same time strangely wonderful. That is just an echo of the tremendous wonder of Divine

Romance. So go ahead: obey the commission— tell your story. Hold hands with the Lover of your soul in public. Become a man after God's own heart!

As you do so, your own bond with His pristine heart will grow stronger. Not only will you be talking about Him, but in some very real and mysterious way, He will begin talking about you! Matthew says it this way: *"Whoever acknowledges me before others, I will also acknowledge before my Father in heaven. But whoever disowns me before others, I will disown before my Father in heaven."* (Matthew 10:32-33 NIV) John the Beloved writes: *"He who overcomes shall be clothed in white garments, and I will not blot out his name from the Book of Life; but I will confess* (acknowledge) *his name before My Father and before His angels."* (Revelation 3:5) That's truly amazing: if you are an overcomer—and that is what this book is inviting you into becoming—then the day will come that Jesus will be talking about your story in the presence of the inner circle of the King of heaven and His private angels. Wow! In a timeless mystery, even as you are practicing His presence, He is practicing yours! Maybe this is what abiding in Christ is all about. (See John 15)

~Assume your governmental position and be fruitful! You have now been seated with Christ in heavenly places (see Ephesians 2:6). And if you are truly turning around and running in a new direction, away from bondage, then your life can now begin to unfold from that heaven-anchored place downward. Your future— believe it!— is now a part of the unstoppable increase of God's government and peace on earth as in heaven. Now that you have stepped into your redemption, you can become fruitful in a lasting, eternal way, like never before. Whereas good works might have previously been a part of the religious process that actually kept you from realizing your tremendous need for intimacy with God in order to combat your depravity, now your intimacy with God frees you to walk in a manner that will overflow in acts of worship and in kindness and love for others in a sincere manner previously inaccessible to you.

The road ahead will be a very personal and unique journey for you and God to walk out in the poetic fragrance of Ephesians 2:10. Overwhelmed and compelled by gratitude for your forgiveness, you have finally been freed to do good works out of true love, rather than as an obligation or out of servitude, or as a means of trying to gain acceptance. (See Luke 7:47)

~Help your brothers! As you continue to move froward in sustained purity, there may be a band of brothers who come alongside of you, men with similar testimonies, similar wounds, similar triumphs. That would be beautiful and may likely happen; but if it does not take place right away, don't worry about it or make it a reason for you to return to the ways of the past. (The old man is dead, remember?) In my journey, I never had a healthy brother commit to help me walk my new line. There were several who could have, and perhaps should have. But instead, when I finally turned the corner on pornographic intimacy, I had God bringing other wounded, diseased brothers to me who also needed help in their walk. I became a part of their rescue. And that in itself lent strength and life and serious import to the maintenance of my own walk with God.

~Control yourself! A most important thing is that you understand that holiness is *your* choice. With the constant help of the Holy Spirit, *you must take full responsibility for all of your actions.* No one else is going to be able to stand before God and answer for your choices. You cannot rely on or depend on someone else to ask you the tough questions, and keep you walking in the light. You have the Holy Spirit, in full measure, living inside of you. Access Him. He must become your combat buddy. Self-control is a fruit of His life inside of you, evidence that you are teamed up and welded together into one inseparable unit. He has freed you to give your will completely to Jesus, moment by moment, day by day, year by year, decade by decade.

~Keep your eyes on eternity! If it helps at all, please know that by faith, I am cheering you on, and fully believing that you and I will meet after the finish line, where it will be my honor to hear *your* story, and how you too became an overcomer. Until that day, keep yourself in the love of God, hidden in His perfect, intimate embrace.

Peace to you. Jeffrey S. Hakes

"Therefore we also, since we are surrounded by so great a cloud of witnesses, let us lay aside every weight, and the sin which so easily ensnares us, and let us run with endurance the race that is set before us, looking unto Jesus, the author and finisher of our faith, who for the joy that was set before Him endured the cross, despising the shame, and has sat down at the right hand of the throne of God." (Hebrews 12: 1-2 NKJV)

Now to Him who is able to
keep you from stumbling,
And to present you faultless
Before the presence of His glory
with exceeding joy,
To God our Savior,
Who alone is wise,
Be glory and majesty,
Dominion and power,
Both now and forever.
Amen. (Jude 24-25)

Appendix A:

Recommended reading

The Bondage Breaker, Neil Anderson

(A youth version of Bondage Breaker—which I have found helpful even for adults for whom reading is more of a challenge—is also available for this book; it is called, Stomping Out the Darkness.)

Healing the Masculine Soul: God's Restoration of Men to Real Manhood, by Gordon Dalbey

Unceasing: an introduction to night and day prayer, by Billy Humphrey

To Know Him: How Intimacy with God Changes Everything, by Billy Humphrey

Red Moon Rising: How Night and Day Prayer is Awaking a Nation, by Pete Grieg

For an excellent resource on sexuality, gender wellness, and related counsel and intercession, please see also: The Broken Image: Restoring Personal Wholeness through Healing Prayer, by Leanne Payne.

Appendix B:

Scriptures for additional meditation:

Psalm 16:11 You will show me the path of life; In Your presence is fullness of joy; at Your right hand are pleasures forevermore.

Psalm 27:4 One thing I have desired of the Lord, that will I seek: that I may dwell in the house of the Lord all the days of my life, to behold the beauty of the Lord, and to inquire in His temple.

Psalm 84:11 For the Lord God is a sun and shield; The Lord will give grace and glory; no good thing will He withhold from those who walk uprightly.

Proverbs 19:23 The fear of the Lord leads to life, and he who has it will abide in satisfaction; he will not be visited by evil.

Luke 17:1-3a Then He said to the disciples, "It is impossible that no offenses should come, but woe to him through whom they do come! It would be better for him if a millstone were hung around his neck, and he were thrown into the sea, than that he should offend one of these little ones. Take heed to yourselves.

Romans 8:1-15 There is therefore now no condemnation to those who are in Christ Jesus, who do not walk according to the flesh, but according to the Spirit. For the law of the Spirit of life in Christ Jesus has made me free from the law of sin and death. For what the law could not do in that it was weak through the flesh, God did by sending His own Son in the likeness of sinful flesh, on account of sin: He condemned sin in the flesh, that the righteous requirement of the law might be fulfilled in us who do not walk according to the flesh but according to the Spirit. For those who live according to the flesh set their minds on the things of the flesh, but those who live according to the Spirit, the things of the Spirit. For to be carnally minded is death, but to be spiritually minded is life and peace. Because the carnal mind is enmity against God; for it is not subject to the law of God, nor indeed can be. So then, those who are in the flesh cannot please God.

But you are not in the flesh but in the Spirit, if indeed the Spirit of God dwells in you. Now if anyone does not have the Spirit of Christ, he is not His. And if Christ is in you, the body is dead because of sin, but the Spirit is life because of righteousness. But if the Spirit of Him who raised Jesus from the dead dwells in you, He who raised Christ from the dead will also give life to your mortal bodies through His Spirit who dwells in you.

Therefore, brethren, we are debtors—not to the flesh, to live according to the flesh. For if you live according to the flesh you will die; but if by the Spirit you put to death the deeds of the body, you will live. For as many as are led by the Spirit of God, these are sons of God. For you did not receive the spirit of bondage again to fear, but you received the Spirit of adoption by whom we cry out, "Abba, Father."

Romans 12:1-2 NCV So brothers and sisters, since God has shown us great mercy, I beg you to offer your lives as a living sacrifice to him. Your offering must be only for God and pleasing to him, which is the spiritual way for you to worship. Do not be shaped by this world; instead be changed within by a new way of thinking. Then you will be able to decide what God wants for you; you will know what is good and pleasing to him and what is perfect.

Romans12:21 Do not be overcome by evil, but overcome evil with good.

Romans 13:11-14 And do this, knowing the time, that now it is high time to awake out of sleep; for now our salvation is nearer than when we first believed. The night is far spent, the day is at hand. Therefore let us cast off the works of darkness, and let us put on the armor of light. Let us walk properly, as in the day, not in revelry and drunkenness, not in lewdness and lust, not in strife and envy. But put on the Lord Jesus Christ, and make no provision for the flesh, to fulfill its lusts.

2 Cor. 5:14-15 For the love of Christ compels us, because we judge thus: that if One died for all, then all died; and He died for all, that those who live should live no longer for themselves, but for Him who died for them and rose again.

2 Cor. 5:16-17 NCV From this time on we do not think of anyone *(especially women)* as the world does . . . If anyone belongs to Christ, there is a new creation. The old things have gone; everything is made new! (emphasis, mine)

2 Cor. 6:14-7:1 . . . what fellowship has righteousness with lawlessness? And what communion has light with darkness? And what accord has Christ with Belial? Or what part has a believer with an unbeliever? And what agreement has the temple of God with idols? For you are the temple of the living God. As God has said: I will be their God, And they shall be My people." Therefore "Come out from among them and be separate, says the Lord. Do not touch what is unclean, and I will receive you." "I will be a Father to you, And you shall be My sons and daughters, Says the Lord Almighty." Therefore, having these promises, beloved, let us cleanse ourselves from all

filthiness of the flesh and spirit, perfecting holiness in the fear of God.

2 Cor. 7:1 ESV Since we have these promises, beloved, let us cleanse ourselves from every defilement of body and spirit, bringing holiness to completion in the fear of God.

Colossians 3:1-7 NCV Since you were raised from the dead with Christ, aim at what is in heaven, where Christ is sitting at the right hand of God. Think only about the things in heaven, not the things on earth. Your old sinful self has died, and your new life is kept with Christ in God. Christ is your life, and when he comes again, you will share in his glory. So put all evil things out of your life: sexual sinning, doing evil, letting evil thoughts control you, wanting things that are evil, and greed. This is really serving a false god. These things make God angry. In your past, evil life you also did these things.

Galatians 5:16-25 I say then: Walk in the Spirit, and you shall not fulfill the lust of the flesh. For the flesh lusts against the Spirit, and the Spirit against the flesh; and these are contrary to one another, so that you do not do the things that you wish. But if you are led by the Spirit, you are not under the law.

Now the works of the flesh are evident, which are: adultery, fornication, uncleanness, lewdness, idolatry, sorcery, hatred, contentions, jealousies, outbursts of wrath, selfish ambitions, dissensions, heresies, envy, murders, drunkenness, revelries, and the like; of which I tell you beforehand, just as I also told you in time past, that those who practice such things will not inherit the kingdom of God.

But the fruit of the Spirit is love, joy, peace, longsuffering, kindness, goodness, faithfulness, gentleness, self-control. Against such there is no law. And those who are Christ's have crucified the flesh with its passions and desires. If we live in the Spirit, let us also walk in the Spirit.

Galatians 6:7-9 Do not be deceived, God is not mocked; for whatever a man sows, that he will also reap. For he who sows to his flesh will of the flesh reap corruption, but he who sows to the Spirit will of the Spirit reap everlasting life. And let us not grow weary while doing good, for in due season we shall reap if we do not lose heart.

Ephesians 3:14-21 For this reason I bow my knees to the Father of our Lord Jesus Christ, from whom the whole family in heaven and earth is named, that He would grant you, according to the riches of His glory, to be strengthened with might through His Spirit in the inner man, that Christ may dwell in your hearts through faith;

that you, being rooted and grounded in love, may be able to comprehend with all the saints what is the width and length and depth and height— to know the love of Christ which passes knowledge; that you may be filled with all the fullness of God.

Now to Him who is able to do exceedingly abundantly above all that we ask or think, according to the power that works in us, to Him be glory in the church by Christ Jesus to all generations, forever and ever. Amen.

1 Timothy 5:1b-2 NIV . . . Treat younger men as brothers, older women as mothers, and younger women as sisters, with absolute purity.

Hebrews 10:26-31 NIV If we deliberately keep on sinning after we have received the knowledge of the truth, no sacrifice for sins is left, but only a fearful expectation of judgment and of raging fire that will consume the enemies of God. Anyone who rejected the law of Moses died without mercy on the testimony of two or three witnesses. How much more severely do you think someone deserves to be punished who has trampled the Son of God underfoot, who has treated as an unholy thing the blood of the covenant that sanctified them, and who has insulted the Spirit of grace? For we know him who said, "It is mine to avenge; I will repay," and again, "The Lord will judge his people." It is a dreadful thing to fall into the hands of the living God.

Hebrew 12:1-3 Therefore we also, since we are surrounded by so great a cloud of witnesses, let us lay aside every weight, and the sin which so easily ensnares us, and let us run with endurance the race that is set before us, looking unto Jesus, the author and finisher of our faith, who for the joy that was set before Him endured the cross, despising the shame, and has sat down at the right hand of the throne of God. For consider Him who endured such hostility from sinners against Himself, lest you become weary and discouraged in your souls.

1 Peter 1:13-17 NIV Therefore, with minds that are alert and fully sober, set your hope on the grace to be brought to you when Jesus Christ is revealed at his coming. As obedient children, do not conform to the evil desires you had when you lived in ignorance. But just as he who called you is holy, so be holy in all you do; for it is written: "Be holy, because I am holy." Since you call on a Father who judges each person's work impartially, live out your time as foreigners here in reverent fear.

1 Peter 1:22 NCV Now that your obedience to the truth has purified your souls, you can have true love for your Christian brothers and sisters. So love each other deeply with all your heart.

1 Peter 3:7 NIV Husbands, in the same way be considerate as you live with your wives, and treat them with respect as the weaker partner and as heirs with you of the gracious gift of life, so that nothing will hinder your prayers.

1 Peter 4:12-13 Beloved, do not think it strange concerning the fiery trial which is to try you, as though some strange thing happened to you; but rejoice to the extent that you partake of Christ's sufferings, that when His glory is revealed, you may also be glad with exceeding joy.

1 Peter 5:8-11 Be sober, be vigilant; because your adversary the devil walks about like a roaring lion, seeking whom he may devour. Resist him, steadfast in the faith, knowing that the same sufferings are experienced by your brotherhood in the world. But may the God of all grace, who called us to His eternal glory by Christ Jesus, after you have suffered a while, perfect, establish, strengthen, and settle you. To Him be the glory and the dominion forever and ever. Amen.

Revelation 21:7-8 He who overcomes shall inherit all things, and I will be his God and he shall be My son. But the cowardly, unbelieving, abominable, murderers, sexually immoral, sorcerers, idolaters, and all liars shall have their part in the lake which burns with fire and brimstone, which is the second death.

Made in the USA
Columbia, SC
07 August 2023